Tibetan Medicine
AND OTHER HOLISTIC
HEALTH-CARE SYSTEMS

Tom Dummer

Tibetan Medicine
AND OTHER HOLISTIC
HEALTH-CARE SYSTEMS

R
ROUTLEDGE
London and New York

First published in 1988 by
Routledge
a division of Routledge, Chapman and Hall
11 New Fetter Lane, London EC4P 4EE

Published in the USA by
Routledge
a division of Routledge, Chapman and Hall, Inc.
29 West 35th Street, New York, NY 10001

Set in Garamond 10 on 12pt
by Columns of Reading
and printed in Great Britain
by The Guernsey Press Co Ltd
Guernsey, Channel Islands

Library of Congress Cataloging in Publication Data
Dummer, Thomas G. (Thomas George)
  Tibetan medicine and other holistic health-care
  systems/Tom Dummer.
    p. cm.
  Bibliography: p.
  Includes index.
  1. Medicine, Tibetan.   2. Therapeutic systems.
  3. Holistic medicine.   I. Title.
  [DNLM: 1. Holistic Health.   2. Medicine, Oriental
  Traditional—China.   WB 50 JC6 D8t]
  R603.T5D86   1988
  610'.9515—dc19
  DNLM/DLC   87–32306

British Library CIP Data also available

ISBN 0–415–01278–3

Contents

PART TWO   Relating Tibetan Medicine to Western Holistic Systems of Medicine

THE DALAI LAMA

F O R E W O R D

Tibetan Medicine is a comprehensive and an
effective system of health care, which over the
centuries has served the Tibetan people well and
we wish to share its great potentialities and
benefits for the health and happiness with all
other peoples in the world.

Until now there has been considerable difficulty
in relating Western systems of medicine to the
traditional medicine of Tibet. The principal
problem has been one of communication.

We hope this book, "Tibetan Medicine" by
Dr. Tom Dummer will help to bridge the gap between
Western and Tibetan medical thinking. Its appearance
is both timely and welcome.

July 27, 1984

This book is dedicated to the Karma-Kagyu Lineage of Tibetan Buddhism, and particularly the 16th Karmapa, Rangjung Rigpe Dorje, whose compassion and concern for all beings was limitless and without bounds.

Acknowledgments

I wish to particularly thank the four outstanding Tibetan medicine teachers and in the case of three of them their excellent and lucid interpreters too – Doctors Trogawa Rinpoche, Yeshi Donden and Tenzin Choedhak. Dr Lobsang Rapgay, a Buddhist monk, in common with many younger generation Tibetans, has an excellent command of English language and idiom. I was therefore able to receive the Teachings direct. Fortunately their presence in the West is on-going at this point in time and long may they continue to visit us and teach.

My warm personal thanks to my friend Mr Gyatsho Tshering, Director of the Library of Tibetan Works and Archives, who has been a constant source of support for this project and full of sound and wise advice.

The Tibetan Medical Institute has been more than helpful since this book was merely a project, from the time of Mr Jigme Tsarong until today with Mrs Namgyal L. Samden-Taklha, the present Director.

I am indebted to both LTWA and TMI who have allowed me to quote freely from the source publicatons of their two organizations. In addition, my many thanks to other authors and particularly Lama Chime Rinpoche, Dr Lobsang Rapgay, the late Terry Clifford, Glen Rein and Marianne Winder, who have allowed me to quote certain passages from their own works and publishers from their publications.

My particular acknowledgments to Marianne Winder. Her expertise concerning Buddhist Texts and the finer points of the

Tibetan language, has been invaluable in ensuring the maximum accuracy of information.

I am very grateful to my old friend of Dharamsala days, Barry Clark who so kindly vetted the whole manuscript. He consequently made a number of constructive suggestions and corrections, which have generally ensured the validity of the information contained herein in respect of the Tibetan medicine aspects.

Thank you Riki Hyde-Chambers and Sam Bercholz for 'twisting my arm' and persuading me to write the book in the first place.

Last, but by no means least, my grateful thanks (a) to Wendy Bedford who has patiently typed and re-typed during the past four years and has never complained once, and (b) James Sumerfield for reading, re-reading, checking and generally ensuring continuity and structure of the final draft.

Tables and Figures

Tables

Figures

Vows of a Tibetan Doctor

1. A person undergoing medical training must have great regard for his Teacher, considering him like a God.

2. He must believe in whatever his Teacher teaches him and have no doubt whatsoever in his teachings.

3. He must have great respect for the books on medicine.

4. He must keep good, friendly relations with classmates, having regard and respect for each other.

5. He must have sympathy towards patients.

6. Secretions of patients he should not regard as filth.

7. He must regard the Medicine Buddha and other medical experts as the guardians of medicine.

8. He must regard medical instruments as holy objects and keep them properly.

9. He must regard medicine as something very precious, something that fulfils all wishes.

10. He must regard medicine as deathless nectar.

11. He must regard medicine as an offering to the Medicine Buddha and all other medicine deities.

Tibetan Medicine, Rechung Rinpoche

Introduction

The 'Land of Snows' – the magic conjured up by these three words is all that exemplifies the old Tibet, so ably and graphically recorded by those outstanding story-tellers, Alexandra David-Neel, Heinrich Harrer and Marco Pallis, to name but a few. Moreover, the folklore and pageantry captures the imagination, the monasteries with their red-robed monks and lamas, the chörtens, the gods, the mountains and demons, the ritual and the mysticism so painstakingly documented by Waddell and other eminent Tibetologists and scholars.

Lhasa, the 'Forbidden City', was the seat of the Dalai Lamas, the spiritual and temporal rulers of Tibet during fourteen incarnations. The Potala, the winter residence, towering high above the city is the legendary abode of Avalokiteshvara (Chenrezig) the patron saint and protector of Tibet, the Great Compassionate One of whom the present Dalai Lama is an emanation. His mantra, OM MANI PADME HUM, is inscribed on thousands upon thousands of mountain surfaces, rocks, 'mani' stones, prayer wheels and flags and was, in the old Tibet, constantly on everyone's lips.

Being brutally ejected in 1959 out of the Middle Ages and into the twentieth century has been a painful and tragic experience for the Tibetan people. But good always comes out of bad, and so much potential good in the form of the rich cultural heritage of Tibet is now available for the first time in the West, at least to those who are prepared to make the effort and acquire some of the untold spiritual wisdom and knowledge which is virtually there for the asking.

Within this context, as an integral part of the Tibetan way of life and culture, the Emchi system of medicine is now, in the West, awaiting our full consideration and investigation. Indeed, although relatively small by comparison with the vast amount of as yet untranslated literature, sufficient is already available in European languages concerning the fundamentals to permit at least a serious study of the subject, if not the full potential application.

Here our thanks go to the amchis (doctors) whose numbers can be counted on both hands, who brought this knowledge with them and, in many cases, as much literature as they could carry, when they left their homeland during some of the most difficult and heroic journeys in the history of refugee migration. For me, whose imagination has always been fired by adventure stories, it was a great moment in my life and, indeed, an honour, to meet personally several years ago Dr Lobsang Dolma, and to learn afterwards from Tibetan friends details of her extraordinary escape across the mountains into India, carrying her two babies on her back together with whatever belongings and 'tools of trade' that she could take with her. Also the dramatic escape of His Holiness The Dalai Lama and the intrepid and daring exploits of the many others who risked their lives, as did Dr Lobsang Dolma, during those dark days of 1959. The story of the refugees' flight from Tibet is told vividly by Chogyam Trungpa Rinpoche in his book *Born in Tibet*.

Writing this book has been an act of faith, as indeed has been my role in the original founding of the Study Group for Tibetan Medicine and my attempts to organize it and maintain it as a valid point of reference for the accumulation and dissemination of knowledge about Tibetan medicine. I am eternally grateful to the few colleagues and friends, Dr Elisabeth Finckh and Miss Marianne Winder, together with Riki Hyde-Chambers of the Tibet Society (UK), who have, all three, sustained my efforts during the past few years. Also to Mr Gyatso Tshering of the Library of Tibetan Works and Archives in Dharamsala and, above all, to His Holiness The Dalai Lama who so graciously agreed to be our patron and who is a constant inspiration to us all.

When it was first suggested that I should write a book on Tibetan medicine particularly with a view to relating it to other forms of medicine, my reaction was totally negative. What could I pretend to know about the subject? Subsequent reflection and talking with friends and colleagues persuaded me to the contrary. Apparently by chance, and certainly not by design, some forty years ago I had found myself as a student of herbal medicine. Again, within the same context of seemingly no choice (my life has always been like that) I served for some fifteen years as the Hon. General-Secretary of IFPNT (International Federation of Practitioners of Natural Therapeutics) where I was in constant contact with the various disciplines of what is now called 'complementary medicine'. I realized that my knowledge of this was considerable. When I think about it, in the light of what I have learned during my relatively brief contact wth Tibetan medicine, I realize that many Western practitioners of other medicines are in a way practising Tibetan medicine through their holistic approaches to healing. Moreover, I'm sure that most of them have never heard of the subject and know little or nothing about the Buddha Dharma.

Although for most of my professional life I have been both practising and teaching osteopathy as a primary therapy, I realize now that my initial training in herbal medicine and my early interest in the healing properties of plants was in fact a 'stepping stone' towards Tibetan medicine. In 1977 I decided to go to India and learn all I could as quickly as possible. My imagination had been fired.

I have heard it said that it takes several lifetimes to become a practitioner of Tibetan medicine. If this is so it would seem that perhaps I am indeed fortunate in already having had at least two lives in one! It is this aspect of Tibetan Buddhism, i.e. karma and rebirth, plus the implied elements of timelessness and familiarity, which have always fascinated me. For instance, when I first set foot in Dharamsala, the hill station in North West India which is now an important Tibetan refugee settlement and headquarters of His Holiness The Dalai Lama and the Tibetan Government in exile, 'Bingo!' that was it! It registered so strongly, the old familiar feeling 'I've been here before'. My mind flashed back to my childhood and I remembered vividly as if it were even today – the birthday present when I was but three years old – the picture book with Tibetan lamas and monks and the monastery with the great shrine room perched on a mountain top! Now I was here in real life, perhaps not with the same mountain top, but certainly with the same mountains before my very eyes. A mere association-reflex, the cynical behaviourist might say. Maybe, but that does not necessarily explain the strong fascination and affinity that, years later, my parents assured me I had for these sights at the age of three. Nor does it fully account for my spontaneous reaction of having been there before and the feeling that I had come home. Karma and rebirth? – who knows!

Constant prodding from colleagues and friends and, particularly, Riki Hyde-Chambers convinced me that I must do what I in the first place had decided was an almost impossible task, i.e. write a book on Tibetan medicine. Hopefully, I have managed to write it in such a way that it will have the widest possible appeal. Finally, bearing in mind that it is such an erudite subject it could so easily end up as a dry-as-dust old tome, I have tried hard to avoid this at all costs, even to the point of being mildly anecdotal. The fact that I am primarily a clinician and not an academic probably weighs in my favour. Indeed, it is my earnest hope that I shall be able to fulfil all the requirements usually demanded of a useful and helpful book. Mercifully it is not solely dealing with the technicalities of Tibetan medicine *per se* and I hope, dear readers, to fire your imaginations and inspire you in the direction of further and far more serious study. If, at the same time, I have presented you with a minimum of factual data so that you will at least be reasonably informed, hopefully entertained, and certainly not bored, then the whole exercise will have been a success and everyone will be happy.

Tom Dummer
London 1986

PART ONE

Traditional Tibetan Medicine

1

Tibetan Medical Philosophy

Historical Origins

A considerable amount of literature on Tibetan medicine already exists in English and other European languages and there are many excellent accounts of its origins, and especially its mythological aspects. With the exception of the reign of one King, Lang Dharma, who banned everything Buddhist, since the 30th King, Srongtsen Gampo, who ruled from the year AD 629–650, Tibet has been a Buddhist country.[1] It was Srongtsen Gampo who introduced Buddhism into Tibet in AD 639, and founded the city of Lhasa. He was also responsible for the written Tibetan alphabet which was adapted from the Sanskrit Devanagarai characters. The consensus of opinion seems to reflect that, while there is evidence that several important forms of medical practice existed in Tibet during the pre-Buddhist era since the seventh century until the present day, Tibetan medicine is found in a purely Buddhist context. As Dr Yeshe Donden has said:

> In ordinary terms Tibetan medicine derives from the Buddha himself, but the actual beginning of our medical system occurred fifty thousand eons ago when it was taught by the Medicine Buddha King. But, indeed, we can say that it came from Sakyamuni Buddha (the historical Buddha) to whom the transmission of the teaching had descended.

The Buddha is said to have manifested as the Medicine Buddha (Men-La). In a thangka-calendar published some years ago by the Tibetan Medical Centre in Dharamsala the central Medicine

3

Buddha is portrayed as Men-la, the medical emanation of Sakyamuni Buddha (Bhaishajaguru), the preceptor of physicians, who is endowed with the beauty and lustre of precious stone — beryl or lapis lazuli. Also known as the Sovereign Healer or the King of Aquamarine Light, he is surrounded by the seven other Medicine Buddhas.

Basic Texts and Commentaries

The Four Medical Tantras form the most important secular work known as the 'Gyu-shi' (rGyud bzhi) which literally means the 'four treatises', viz.: the Root Treatise or Mula Tantra (rtsa-rgyud); the Explanatory Text — Akhyata Tantra (bShad-rgyud); the Practice Instruction Text — Upadesha Tantra (man-ngag-rgyud), being detailed instruction on practice; and the Last Text (appendices) — Uttantra (phyi-ma-rgyud) which is an explanatory account of the other three Tantras.

Written in the form of questions and answers between the great Rishi Rig-Pa'i Yeshes and Rishi Yid-las-skye, both emanations of the Medicine Buddha, this work has four sections, 156 chapters and 5900 verses. Dr Bhagwan Dash[2] says that some portions of the rGyud bzhi are so identical with certain Ayurvedic classics that it can be safely said that one is a translation of the other. Although it was thought that the Sanskrit original of the rGyud bzhi was probably written around AD 400, there are now only Tibetan and Mongolian translations in existence, the latter having been translated from the former. The Tibetan translation is generally attributed to Vairocana who took it from India to the Tibetan King Tri-song Detsan (755–97). His Royal Court physician, Yuthog Yontan Gonpo the Elder, not only edited it, but also wrote the eighteen supplements to it. Later his emanation, Yuthog Yontan Gonpo the Younger, re-edited it. It is generally agreed that this is the version in use today. Indeed, according to one source, Yuthog the Younger was Rishi Rig Pa Yeshe and Sumthon Yeshi, Yuthog's favourite disciple, was Rishi Yid-las-skye.

Elisabeth Finckh quotes Unkrig, who casts doubt on the original and generally accredited authorship. According to another less religiously orientated translation, he says, the original Sanskrit manuscipt was written by Kumarajivaka, the famous Indian physician and contemporary of Sakyamuni, the historical Buddha.[3]

Be that as it may, Dr Yeshe Donden says that Kumarajivaka in any case received the Teachings from the Buddha, therefore the rGyud bzhi is the standard basic work on Tibetan medicine in which all the rules and procedures for its practice are laid down. The published works of Dr Elisabeth Finckh in Europe and Doctors Y. Donden, P. Dorje and L. Champei, Messrs G. Tshering, T.G. Tsarong, J.G. Drakton and Kelsang in Dharamsala provide comprehensive and meticulous translations and schematic tables for the aspiring Western student of the principal and most important parts of the rGyud bzhi and other literature.[4]

According to Dr Bhagwan Dash[5] there are many commentaries on this work but the most important are: 'Legs-bsad Nor-bu' by Byang-pa (fourteenth century); the fourteenth-century commentary by Zur-mkharba in Nyan-nyid rDorje; Vaidurya Sngon-po (Blue Lapis Lazuli) by sDe-srid Sangs-rgyas-rGa-mtsho.

Concerning other important medical texts belonging to the pre-Buddhist era, in India, for example, it is said that just as the Buddha Kasyapa taught medicine in a past aeon, the historical Buddha, Sakyamuni, the fourth of a thousand Buddhas in this Kalpa, 2500 years ago in India, after delivering his first sermon in Sarnath (near Benares), taught the medical text called Vimalagotra. Buddha also taught, when turning the third wheel of the Dharma, the medical text shel gyi me-long (Crystal Mirror). He also gave the teaching of gCer-mthong rigpa'i rGyud to Sariputra and Ananda, his foremost disciples, which consists of 3500 chapters dealing with body hygiene, health and disease, causes and prevention, dietary rules, etc. Asvaghosha also figured importantly at the time of Nagarjuna and wrote the Yan-lag brgyad-pa chen-po[6] with eight great branches of medicine, two complementary texts and a commentary.

There are also within this context a group of medical texts attributed to various Mahabodhisattvas which teach the Bodhisattva methods:

1. Chenrezigs (Bodhisattva Avalokiteshvara) text on general surgery.
2. Jampalyang (Bodhisattva Manjushri) texts on the treatment of head injuries and surgery.

3. Channa Dorje (Bodhisattva Vajrapani) treatise on anatomy.
4. Dolma (Bodhisattva Tara) 120 chapters on herbs and medicinal plants.

Apart from the works and authors briefly mentioned here, there are many others pertinent to Tibetan medicine which derive from the time of the historical Buddha and over a period of 2500 years until the present day. For instance, Guru Rinpoche (Padmasambhava)[7] wrote an important text called bDud-rtsi'i sNying-po (Nectar Essence) as well as other medical works. For historical completeness please refer to the appropriate literature.[8]

In common with all Tibetan Vajrayana texts (Secret Mantrayana), Tibetan medical texts appear to be no exception in their cryptic nature and the deliberate system of camouflage. The purpose of this is to prevent exploitation by persons who might abuse the knowledge contained therein. Commentaries on texts, however, provide a means whereby the deeper and more subtle aspects may be understood. For only those with a profound grasp of the Tibetan language can hope to fully appreciate directly the meaning of the texts in depth.

Regarding the contribution of other countries apart from India to the founding and evolution of Tibetan medicine as such, since King Srongtsen Gampo in the seventh century convened the first international medical conference in Asia, those eminent physicians and important texts from China, Mongolia, Persia, Ladakh and Nepal have been of fundamental importance. It is also said that an important Greek influence came to bear and that Plato may even have visited Tibet.[9]

There is an amusing paradox concerning the Chinese aspect, cited by Dr Yeshi Donden,[10] who says that although Chinese medicine had an undoubted influence on Tibetan medicine, the science of ser-khab or 'golden needle' healing originated first in Tibet and did not derive originally, as is generally supposed, from Chinese acupuncture. It is stated in the 'gSo-rig Chojung' (History of Medical Science), that Mongolian scholars learnt the science of acupuncture from the Tibetan amchis and they in turn imparted it to the Chinese. Ironically, as acupuncture became more popular in China its practice declined in its homeland, Tibet.

The first school of Tibetan medicine was established by the 5th

Dalai Lama at Ganden Monastery. Later a medical college and hospital was built near Lhasa at Chagpori. During the reign of the 13th Dalai Lama a new college of Astrology and Medicine was built at Lhasa, called sMan-rtsis-khan, where Dr Yeshi Donden trained in the 1930s.

The development of Tibetan medicine actually took place in three phases. Firstly, in the Deva world. In Tibetan mythology[11] it began with Brahma who first heard the teaching from Buddha Kasyapa. Brahma composed the gSo-dpyad 'Bum-pa ('1000 verses on Medicine') and it was then passed on to Indra through various Deva-Rishis and ultimately to the King of Benares, coming to be known as the Divine Brahma System of Medicine, the first in the world of men. It also included the Bodhisattva methods referred to above. Secondly, its development during the pre-Tibetan period in India, principally involving Sakyamuni Buddha, Vairochana, Asvahagosha, Aryadeva, Kumarajiva, Shantideva, etc. Thirdly, came the actual development of the science of medicine in Tibet itself with Yuthog Yontan Gonpo (the Elder and Younger), Rinchen Zangpo, Bu-Ston, Sangye Gyatso and so up to the present day with Doctors Yeshi Donden, Lobsang Dolma, Tenzin Choedhak, the Ven. Trogawa Rinpoche, Lobsang Rapgay and Lobsang Wangyal.

Apart from the influence in the development of Tibetan medicine of medical knowledge from India, China, Mongolia, Nepal and Ladakh, the influence of Bön, the indigenous religion, has been important. As Dr Bhagwan Dash[12] says:

The earliest inhabitants of the pre-Buddhist era probably practised shamanism, which was prevalent in the whole of Northern Asia, the Tibetan form of this being known as the Bön religion.

This still exists today, notably in the Tibetan medical/cultural system as it is practised by the Newars and Tibetans in Nepal, i.e. the system of ceremonial medicine, where the Bön influence is strongly in evidence. Accordingly to Dr Bhagwan Dash, the four works on medicine based on the Bön religious tradition, which have been more recently published by the Tibetan Bönpo Monastic Centre (1972), provide ample evidence of Ayurveda in that medical tradition.[13]

2

Buddhist Tantra, Cosmology and Symbolism Relevant to Tibetan Medicine

Since the philosophy of Tibetan medicine is Buddhist, different aspects of the Dharma constantly re-emerge throughout the whole of this book, inasmuch as they are pertinent to the subject matter of each chapter. Therefore, certain repetition is inevitable to illustrate the relevant themes in context. Where more detail is found regarding certain topics in the chapters concerned, only simple reference and definition is included here. The many facets of Buddhist Tantra, cosmology and symbolism are described in considerable detail and in fascinating style by Lama Govinda and Detlef Ingo Lauf.[1]

Tantra

The word Tantra literally means 'lineage' and is used in relation to Buddhism in two ways:

1. To imply continuity in terms of cause and effect, or as the Ven. Trungpa Rinpoche has expressed it — within this context there is continuity of being with a point of departure and a direction — Tantra involves the immediate human situation arising out of how we are going to be in terms of relationship to something or someone. And again, in a practical sense, 'Tantra is a way of inner growth, it makes us see more, so that we really become individuals rather than mere entities.'[2]

2. When referring to the classification of the higher esoteric
Teachings of the Buddha (Shakyamuni), i.e. the Tantras.

Tantric Buddhism often utilizes in its symbolism the male/
female energy principle – deity and consort in union, expressing
compassion and skilful means on the one hand and wisdom on the
other. Despite a multiplicity of non-sexual meanings Tantric
symbolism has been regarded as highly suspect within the context
of those ingrained Western attitudes which take a very negative
approach to sexuality. Guenther[3] expresses it nicely:

> The main charge levelled against Tantrism is that it makes use
> of sex. As is well known, sexual imagery is excluded from
> religious symbolism in the West, while erotic forms are freely
> used in the East for conveying religious feelings. Sex has no evil
> associations for a follower of the Tantras. But this does not
> imply licentiousness.

One sultry afternoon strolling around in Durbar Marg in
Kathmandu, I felt myself being drawn towards a thangka and curio
stall. As I drew nearer, the poor quality of the obviously fake
thangkas became more than evident. However, one was conspic-
uous inasmuch as its curtain was down. With a salacious, toothless
grin the vendor gave a deft and decidedly theatrical tweak to the
curtain and all was revealed – 'Oh look sir the gods are having
sex'. Influenced no doubt by a mixture of intuition and empirical
appreciation of Western prurience, his sales technique was direct
and dramatic. No doubt it was not entirely lost on the
considerable tourist traffic in Kathmandu. This of course is just
what Tantra is *not*.

In conclusion it may be said that Tantra means fully experienc-
ing life without being involved,[4] attached or identified with the
Five Poisons, i.e. the five negative states of ignorance, aggression-
hatred; passion; pride and envy, all of which ultimately depend on
attachment (clinging and grasping). Without attachment, no new
karma is created and accumulated. In spiritual development this
equates with the seventh bodhisattva bhumi (level) –
darsanamarga. One level of karmic concretion (klesavarana) is
removed one at a time at each of the first seven levels (bhumis).

At the level of the Eighth Bhumi – Acala – the remaining three are removed so that Bodhisattva is entirely free from klesavarana. These defilements are all removed by meditation on the Void (Sunyata). No new karma is created and all the old has gone. When all levels are realized Buddha mind is obtained. (See page 31 – the Bodhisattva.) The Five Poisons ultimately become the Three which in their turn identify with the Three Humours (Chapter 3).

Prana, the Psychic Channels and the Cakras

Prana (Skt), ch'i (Chinese) is Life-Force Energy, rLung (Tibetan) or Wind. The nadis or rtsa represent a network of psychic channels – 84,000 in all – through which there is, or should be, a continuous circulation of prana (Wind) if Homeostasis and health are to be maintained. Tobacco smoke is notorious for blocking the nadis. Prana is envisaged as being the total potential energy of mind and body and the dynamic forces formed by the five cosmophysical energies of earth, water, fire, air and space. As we shall see later if these five energies (or elements) become imbalanced, disturbances of what are known as the Three Humours (which correspond to the Three Poisons) will occur, giving rise to various states of ill health. A fuller explanation of the psychic channels and body energies within a Tibetan medical context follows.

The Psychic Channels and Body-Energies within a Tibetan Medicine Context

In Tibetan medicine, as Dr Lobsang Rapgay has pointed out, the body is considered on different levels. For instance on the more gross level it is divided into five areas and each one correlates with a Buddha Family and a particular type of energy, viz.:–

Buddha Vairocana – energy corresponds with the head
Buddha Amitabha – energy corresponds with the neck and throat
Buddha Akshobya – energy corresponds with the thorax and heart

Buddha Ratnasambhava – energy corresponds with the lower abdomen
Buddha Amoghasiddhi – energy corresponds with the limbs and genitals
(Please refer to Tables 1 and 2 in this chapter)

In Tibetan massage for instance, it is within these areas one searches manually for specific tension.

In Maitri or Space Therapy as devised by the Ven. Trungpa Rinpoche,[5] each Buddha family reflects basic styles of relating to space. Typically associated neuroses specific in pattern to the Ego's efforts to relate to space (the world outside in this instance) produce equally typical patterns of neurotic suffering, which may if unresolved lead to actual psychosis. This is involving the more psychological level of course. The more gross Five-Element levels together with the very subtle Essence levels and those of the psychic-channels, etc., figure enormously in both Buddhist spiritual practice and Tantric healing or Dharmic medicine.[6]

The Psychic Channels

The complex system of nadis (tsta) are sometimes referred to in the vernacular as the 'race-track'. This is because the mind (or consciousness) is carried on the 'horse' of prana (vital energy).

The spinal column, apart from its anatomical and physiological role as the central focus of the musculo-skeletal system, microcosmically is also the 'axis-mundi' (see Chapter 2 – 'Mount Meru') which identifies with the central channel (or median nerve) or the Nadi – Uma. There are in all 84,000 channels, some carrying energy, some blood, and others carrying both.

The central-channel distributes to twenty-four main channels which subdivide into seventy-two smaller channels. The Mother White channel, which originates in the brain, descends via the spinal column and is involved in various physiological functions, particularly the motor-nervous. For example, if a blockage or interference occurs within the Mother White channel there can be grave consequences for motor functions. 'Nerves', said Dr Choedhak, 'start in the brain.' There are also six other white channels which are derived from the Mother White channel and

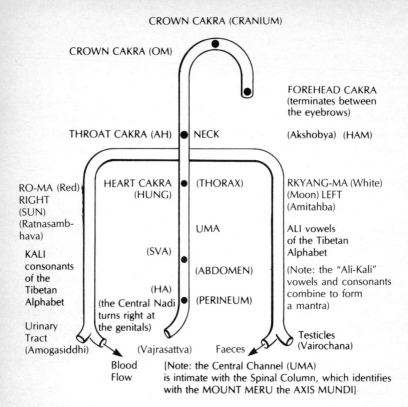

Figure 1 *The Central Channels (Nadis) and correspondences with the Five Jinas*

which originate in the hind-brain, three on each side of the body which are also descending. White channels are generally downward-going from the brain, but there is also an upward-going channel originating from the back of the liver, which carries blood. This is known as the 'principal blood vein'.

All Wind channels connect up with all organs and functions, and two energy channels particularly innervate the heart and intestines. Another energy channel arises in the tella surcica and also innervates the heart plus the lungs, and there is another important one to the reproductive system. Each side of the central channel (Uma), whose function aids also in haemopoiesis, are two other main Wind channels. To the right Ro-ma and to the left Rkyang-ma. Ro-ma is associated with the sun, is red in colour and identifies with Fire and the male genes. Rkyang-ma is associated with the moon, is white in colour, and identifies with Water and the female genes. These, together with the bindu (thig-le), are visualized in certain meditational and yogic practices. There are twenty-four main veins and arteries of which the spinal artery (the aorta) is the most important. In addition, there are twenty-four main veins and arteries which go from the abdomen to the head. One assumes that these could correlate with the twenty-four moveable vertebrae. There are also eight blood vessels which ascend from the lower part of the body to the upper. They then branch out and descend again to the lower structures. All blood vessels contain Wind channels, for it is the Wind energy which circulates the blood, which in its turn goes everywhere. From the 7th vertebra there is a vein to the liver, from the 11th a vein to the gall-bladder and another from the 14th to the kidneys. Similarly there are veins to all twelve major organs.

There is a particular channel – the heart channel – which carries a mixture of blood and energy. There are four connections within the heart. In 'Listening' to the pulse one 'tunes in', says Dr Choedhak,[7] to these four beating veins of the heart, by palpating the radial artery, the carotid artery, the femoral artery in the leg and in the abdomen (inguinal region). In other words pulses can be taken at all these points. The beats arise of course because of the combination of energy and blood flow. This is also responsible for the palpable phenomena associated with Tibetan pulse diagnosis.

There are also four White Phlegm channels. All these connect up with all organs and are associated with the control of the physiological functions of the body, in terms of energy, fluidity and heat.

To conclude this brief description of the psychic channels starting at the central meridian point (near the Inion or occipital protuberance) there are:

4 rLung (Wind) energy channels
4 mKhris-pa (Bile) energy channels
4 Bad-kan (Phlegm) energy channels

which also go to the viscera or body organs. In addition, blood channels run from the lower body to the upper, and nerve channels from the upper to the lower. This arrangement represents a meeting of the male and female principle, i.e. in expressing both polarity and balance.

In conclusion, it would seem that when listening to Tibetan doctors there is some ambiguity concerning the words 'nerves' and 'veins' – for instance: White Nerves; Red Blood Vessels. At one point I felt that there was almost an inexplicable vagueness. The problem is now solved, indeed Keith Dowman elucidates clearly in *Sky Dancer* (p. 246). As he says, the word nadi (rtsa) is the same one whether it be referring to physical – veins, arteries, sinews, tendons or muscles – or indeed the psychic channels themselves. In a similar omnibus way, wind, breath, vital energy, nervous energy, mental energy are all encompassed in the meaning of the word – rLung – Wind. This of course is a clear example of the difficulties that can arise when communication is attempted between persons of two distinct philosophical conditioning, culture and outlook. This also explains why Tibetan medical teachings and explanations are sometimes difficult for Westerners to comprehend. One is equally reminded of the inordinate difficulty encountered in some of the early translations of the Pali Canon. The totally unsatisfactory translation of the word 'Dukka' is a case in point.

Cakras* (Khorlo)

Cakras are the various psychic centres which are of lotus formation. Each lotus has a different number of petals. The five principal centres are situated on the central channel and are connected with the psychic channels generally at the following levels: cranium, throat, heart, navel and perineum. The various correspondences will be seen in Table 1.

The Trikaya (Skt)

(Kaya means body, Tri means Three). The Doctrine of the Three Bodies of the Buddha, Detlef Ingo Lauf[8] writes: 'The three bodies

---

* pronounced 'chakra'

together encompass all the possibilities of Being between the highest Being in the spiritual sense and the objective existence in the world of form'. The Three Bodies are known as the:

(a) Dharmakaya
(b) Sambhogakaya
(c) Nirmanakaya

A fourth Body, Svabhavikakaya, is an experiential unity in perfection of all Three.

Lama Chime Rinpoche[9] describes these three levels of existence succinctly:

The three categories of Tantric teaching
(A) *Dharmakaya*[10]

    (i) is the origin and ground of everything – it has no beginning and no end – it is beyond the limitation and partiality of description – the infinite and formless Reality that Saykamuni Buddha realized.

    (ii) it is also the Universal Mind, that by which everything knows and which knows in anything. But this awareness is not limited in any way and does not know in terms of subject and object. It knows throughout reality; there is nothing other than it which knows.

    (iii) is also the Infinite Void, without form, without sign of termination of any sort, an infinite reservoir beyond distinctions of time and space, not a void in the sense of an absence excluding existence, but a void so without qualities that it can include everything.

    (iv) it is the play of the Universal Mind within the Infinite Void, an inconceivable dynamism never departing from itself, an infinite potentiality and source of freedom and energy, which is limitless.

(B) *Sambhogakaya*

    (i) The first limitation of this infinity takes place on this level. Instead of being fully conditioned within itself, it makes a centre, turns and radiates outwards in a four-fold pattern.

(ii) one aspect of the Sambhogakaya is the Mandala of the 5 WISDOMS — described in the Tantric Mahayana. They are not arbitrary creations of the imagination, but show the primordial nature of the emanation of the Sambhogakaya.

(iii) at the same time, with the separation from the Dharmakaya, Mind turns back upon itself and becomes a specialized womb with the Universal Void: from this we have the creation of fullness and emptiness, positive and negative, a going with the source or turning away from it. The limited space of mind permits only a limited play, and gives rise to the four processes symbolized by the elements — air, fire, earth and water; movement, radiance, expansion and contraction (centrifugal and centripetal).

(iv) all these aspects of the Sambhogakaya are summed up in the Mandala of the FIVE JINAS or DYHANI-BUDDHAS. Each Buddha is related to a direction in space and to one of the elemental processes.

(v) each Dyhani-Buddha has an aspect of ignorance which proceeds from the coming into existence of DUALITY, which in company with his consort, he neutralizes and overcomes.

(vi) the visualization of a Buddha of a particular form or colour is only the first step; the form and colour is however the one most appropriate; it is the Nirmanakaya form of that particular wisdom and so it can act as a link. When the real Dyhani-Buddha is understood, then the knowledge, wisdom and power necessary to overcome one form of ignorance is found.

The Sambhogakaya level cannot be directly perceived by the senses, since it is the *Energy* Level, but nevertheless can be subtly sensed or appreciated. Sambhogakaya manifestation is not visible through normal sensory appreciation. Several examples however come to mind. Only those of sufficient spiritual development are able to see the actual Vajra Crown of the Karmapas, i.e. the Sambhogakaya version which was made originally of an unknown substance by the Dakinis — not, of course, the Nirmanakaya material-form Vajra Crown which is worn by the Gyalwa Karmapas during the Black Hat ceremony. Another example, from the Bible, concerns the Ascension. Certain of the Disciples were able to see Christ's 'glorified body' which was a Sambhogakaya manifestation, but others not so spiritually advanced were able to see only His Nirmanakaya body.

(C) *Nirmanakaya*

    (i) From the Sambhogakaya comes the Nirmanakaya, the CREATION OF INDIVIDUAL BEINGS WITH FORM. Each aspect of the Sambhogakaya expresses itself within the Nirmanakaya. The 5 Wisdoms are expressed as the 5 constituents of personality.

    (ii) the 5 Skandas — knowing, willing, thought and sensation, feeling and form. Each of the 5 Jinas (Dhyani-Buddhas) is related to one of these, and through them it may be purified and reach harmony and enlightenment.

    (iii) from the coming into existence of POSITIVE and NEGATIVE comes the DUALITY which runs through existence — of SEPARATION FROM THE SOURCE and RETURNING TO THE SOURCE.

    (iv) in the course of nature the opposites can work smoothly e.g. night and day, growing and dying etc. But because there has been separation into individual beings, an individual can choose to prolong his period of separation beyond the overall harmony of the Sambhogakaya pattern; *that* is ignorance (avidja)* and the creation of suffering (dukkha).†
Ignorance and suffering are not inevitable in the Nirmanakaya, they are just likely. In practice, however, most beings in this particular world have chosen them.

    (v) all actions, good or bad, all thoughts, everything that is done enters the womb of this DUALITY and

---

* Pali: avijyā   † Pali: dukkha
Sanskrit: avidyā   Sanskrit: duhka

constitute ALAYA-VIJNANA (or store-consciousness), by which the pattern of the present is produced out of the past, and so on.

(vi) the Sambhogakaya forces enter and create the patterns of the Nirmanakaya:
- species – nations,
- womb and egg,
- brother and sister,
- tide and orbit, etc.

THIS CONTINUES UNTIL THE PURPOSES OF DUALITY ARE FULFILLED AND EXHAUSTED.

(vii) The FORM and ENERGY that is required by the Nirmanakaya come from the PRIMORDIAL ELEMENTAL PROCESES: i.e. the FIVE ELEMENTS or cosmo-physical Energies:

(a) SPACE gives the STARTING POINT.
(b) AIR gives movement and dynamism.
(c) FIRE gives energy and heat.
(d) EARTH gives extension (expansion) through growth.
(e) WATER gives cohesion (contraction) necessary for form.

BY BALANCING THESE FORCES AT ALL LEVELS WITHIN A BODY ONE CAN ENSURE ITS HARMONY AND HEALTH.

Conclusion (Chime Rinpoche)

These 3 Bodies are not separate in reality; they are a UNITY. The complete body which they compose is called the *AKASHDHATU*.

In that sense a being can continue to 'exist' even though he has reached enlightenment and no longer needs to exist in the ordinary sense. His existence can be infinite, it can work in form at the same time. He is not limited by causality, but is free to create his own causality and movement through the universe in harmony with the whole.

The Five Elements (Cosmo-physical energies)

In Chapter 3 the fundamental role of the Five Elements forming the basis of all phenomena associated with Tibetan medicine is expanded upon. Meantime it can be mentioned that three levels of Five-Element manifestation are described, the:

1. gross element, and
2. subtle element levels, and
3. essence of the element level.

The Relevance of the Subtle Energies to Healing

Thinley Norbu[11] describes in great detail and completeness both the horizontal, vertical and the ultimately 'total interdependence' manifestation on all levels pertaining to all dualistic samsaric phenomena, plus the mental yoga by which they may be rebalanced, harmonized and resolved into non-dualistic emptiness, in terms of Dzog-chen, the spiritual method of the Great Perfection according to Higher Yoga Tantra.

His views on healing generally and, in particular, his advice to doctors are tantamount to being the last words on the subject – indeed, the ultimate expression in healing of the Great Perfection. Those doctors and practitioners who are able to follow and truly apply this advice stand to find clinical results considerably enhanced. Moreover, the resulting improvements in health will be seen to be emanating from a deeper and more fundamental level within the patients concerned.

Basically, as Thinley Norbu points out, unless the doctor or practitioner's mind is able to appreciate and apply itself on the subtle essence of the element level, the resulting treatment will only be effective relative to the conceptual level of the practitioner's mind itself. The rebalancing process will only be either partially and/or superficially complete, the clinical result only symptomatic and partial and most probably only temporary. Diagnosis is equally either incomplete and symptomatic as opposed to being fundamental and correct, because the doctor's mind is able to perceive only the interplay of the gross elements and/or at the best the subtle element level, but unable to appreciate — let alone give direct help to — the patient on the essence of the element level. This ancient Tantric 'Wisdom Mind' view has its direct contemporary parallel in Western osteopathic medicine, as originally described and practised by the great pioneers A.T. Still and W.G. Sutherland (see Chapter 14).

The Five Jinas

As previously mentioned, the five principal centres are situated on the central channel and it is within these that the Five Jinas are seated. In addition to the association of the Five Jinas (Dhyani Buddhas) with the Five Cakras, they are also identified with the Four Medical Tantras. Thus it was said that when the Buddha manifested the medicine mandala, He emitted *five* rays of light from his *five* secret points to the five Jinas accordingly. Seated at the throat cakra, which is associated with the faculty of speech, is Buddha Amitabha who has the role of acting as the intermediary, i.e. to request the Teachings on the Four Medical Tantras as follows:

Buddha Vairocana   — associated with the activity of the body, is seated at the crown cakra and is responsible for the Teaching of the 2nd Tantra, which incidentally treats principally with the embryology, anatomy and physiology.

Buddha Akshobyha   — associated with the activity of Mind, is seated at the heart cakra, is responsible for the Teaching of the 1st Tantra — the Root Treatise, the fundamentals.

Buddha Ratnasambhava — associated with the activity of Merit, is seated at the navel cakra, is responsible for the Teaching of the 3rd Tantra. Principally pathology and disease classification.

Buddha Amoghasiddhi — associated with the activity of Deeds (Karma), is seated at the perineum cakra, is responsible for the Teaching of the 4th Tantra, concerned with actual clinical practice.

The Five Jinas are also, in a medical context, referred to as the Five Rishis. Holism and relativity are thus, by such arrangements and concepts, symbolically expressed.

The Five Buddha Families

The Five Buddha Families (in the Tantras) originally thought of as being six, i.e. the Five plus Vajrasattva, express the Five Buddha Energies — Buddha, Ratna, Padma, Karma and Vajra. A contemporary therapeutic application of this has been evolved by the Ven. Trungpa Rinpoche — Maitri therapy.

In the evolution of the idea, the Five Buddha Families and Energies are reduced in combination to Three — the Vajras of body, speech and mind.

Buddha Ratna	Vajra of body (Kaya)
Padma Karma	Vajra of speech (Vac)
Aksobhya + Vajrasattva	Vajra of mind (Citta)

In a vertical sense the Five Cakras correspond to all the groups of five to be found in Table 1, which gives a few of the correspondences to illustrate the general idea. The various horizontal correspondences — Dharmic, anatomical, physiological, psychological-behavioural — particularly relevant to Tibetan medicine are shown in Table 2, together with a key for reference purposes. These are probably no more than a third or perhaps a half of the groupings of *five* found in Tantric Buddhism which go to make up the total cosmological view of the whole of existence.

Table 1 Some correspondences of the Five Cakras

Cakra	Colour	Bija	Jina	Element
head	white	OM	Vairocana	Space
throat	red	AH	Amitahba	Fire
heart	blue	HUM	Akshobhya	Water
navel	yellow	SVA	Ratnasambhava	Earth
perineum	green	HA	Amogasiddhi	Air

Mount Meru

Mount Meru is the mythical 'axis mundi' of the four continents as symbolized in the mandala of the universe. Mount Meru is identified with Mount Kailash in Tibet and also the spinal column in *homo sapiens*.

The Medicine Buddha sMan-lha (Men-la)

It is said that the Buddha, when he appeared as the Medicine Buddha, spent four years in LTa-Na-sdug (Tanaduk), a mythical mountain plateau city (see Chapter 10). This, again, is said to be the same place as Indra's Palace on Mount Meru and where He taught the rGyud bzhi. Various Buddhas and Deities have their own particular Buddhafields (or heavens). In the mandala of the Five Jinas, the Buddhafield of sMan-gyi-rgyal-po (Men-La), the Medicine Buddha, is said to be situated further east, far out but in the same direction from the realm of Akshobhya/Vairocana. Moreover, there are seven other Buddhafields for the seven other Medicine Buddhas:

1. Sha'-kya-thub-pa;
2. gSer-bzang dri-med;

cont. on p. 26

Table 2 Correspondences relevant to Tibetan medicine

	Vairocana (Buddha)	Amitabha (Padma)	Aksobhya (Vajra)	Ratnasambhava (Ratna)	Amogasiddhi (Karma)
1.					
2.	Cakra	Padme (Lotus)	Vajra	Ratna	Vishvajra
3.	white (Dhatu: blue)	red	blue (Dhatu: white)	yellow	green
4.	centre (zenith and nadir)	West	East	South	North
5.	OM	AH	HUM	SVA	HA
6.	dharmacakra	meditation	earth-touching	giving	fear-dispelling
7.	lion	peacock	elephant	horse	garuda
8.	dharmadhatu	discriminating	mirror like	equanimity	all-performing
9.	ignorance, mental confusion, delusion	passion/lust	hatred and aggression	pride and slander	envy, jealousy and paranoia
10.	Space	Fire	Water	Earth	Air

Table 2 *cont.*

	spring	winter	autumn	summer
11.	—	—			
12.	—	dusk – sunset	dawn – sunrise	day – noon	night
13.	consciousness (Vijnana)	perceptions related to discriminating awareness (Samjna)	form, body consciousness (Rupa)	feelings, emotion (Vedana)	intellect, concepts, will, ideas, personality, motivation (Samskara)
14.	taste	sight	hearing	smell	touch
15.	—	facade, lack of depth, superficial	texture	depth	consistency, workableness
16.	head	neck and throat	thorax and heart	lower abdomen	limbs and genitals
17.	eyes	nose	torso – skin	ears	tongue
18.	faeces	urine	semen	blood	flesh (human)
19.	Metal	Fire	Water	Earth	Wood

20.	crown/forehead (Head Centre)	throat	heart	navel	perineum
21.	grief	sympathy	anger	joy	fear
22.	sloth and torpor	senility	aversion	scepticism	worry
23.	astringent	hot	bitter	sweet	salty
24.	forms	odours	tangibles	sounds	tastes
25.	body	speech	mind	merits	acts

KEY

1. Jina Buddha Family and Energy
2. Symbol and Energy
3. Colour
4. Direction
5. Bija Mantra
6. Mudra
7. Animal or Bird
8. Wisdom
9. Klesa or Mental Poison
10. Element
11. Season
12. Time
13. Skandha
14. Sense
15. Quality
16. Anatomical correspondence
17. Sense Organs
18. Five Amrtas (Ambrosias)
19. Five Elements (pulses)
20. Cakras
21. Emotions
22. Five Hindrances to practising the Dharma
23. Five Tastes (or flavours)
24. Five Knowables
25. Five Superintendencies

3. sGra-dbyang rgyal-po;
4. Chos-grags rgya-mtsho;
5. Mya-ngan-med-mchog;
6. mNgon mkhyen rgyal-po;
7. mTsan-legs yongs-grags.[6]

The Medicine Buddha is sometimes depicted holding a myrobalan fruit or sprig from the tree. This fruit, in Tibetan, is 'dug-bcom', which means 'that which renders poison inactive'. As a symbol of the healing art it is called 'dug-sel', 'that which expels poison'. A spiritual connotation is included in the word poison, e.g. the Three Poisons, attachment or aversion, hatred and ignorance or close-mindedness, as well as reference to the obvious material-physical poisons (toxins). Dr Yeshi Donden again emphasizes what has been said before – that attachment, in the form of clinging and grasping, dominates the other poisons.

The Triratna (Three Jewels)

Basic Buddhism (Theravadin) teaches that the Three Jewels are:

1. The Buddha – the historical Buddha Shakyamuni;
2. The Dharma – the Teachings of the Buddha;
3. The Sangha – the company of monks, i.e. those who have renounced the worldly life.

Mahayana Buddhism teaches a wider and more comprehensive understanding:

1. That of many Buddhas all emanating from the Adibuddha (the historical Buddha Shakyamuni being the fourth of 1000 Buddhas in this Kalpa).
2. The Teachings of the Buddha to include the Sutras.
3. The Sangha – not only the brethren of the cloth, but all those 'spiritual companions' (Kalyānamitra) who have formally taken commitment-vows.

Vajrayana Buddhism, which is basically the Mahayana model but which includes the third of the Buddha's Teachings — the Tantras — has evolved a further triad, the Three Roots:

1. Lama — the guru, the spiritual guide who confers initiation on the Dharma student.
2. Yidam — the personal meditative and protective deity of the initiate.
3. Dakini — she is the 'wise-one' who transmits the secret wisdom to the initiate through the 'inner voice'.

The Four Kayas and the Six Realms (Including the Tibetan Wheel of Life)

Body (Kaya), speech (Vacca) and mind (Citta) are for *homo sapiens* the three modes of existence which in the final analysis are interdependent and interrelated as one in the individual human personality. The aberrations of body, speech and mind determine the karma of both the present life and of rebirth.

The Three Poisons (dug-gsum) relate and identify with body, speech and mind, which in their turn identify with the brow, throat and heart cakras, the bijas — OM, AH, HUM — and the colours white, red and blue respectively.

1. Attachment/Clinging — originates at the level of the active intellect and desire, and manifests in the forehead cakra.
2. Hatred/Aversion — expresses itself in speech and manifests in the throat cakra.
3. Ignorance and Spiritual Darkness — is associated with the heart cakra (the level of the Awareness Mind).

By initiation all negative mental contaminations and aberrations (the Five and Three Poisons) are neutralized or, better still, removed, and all the positive virtues and clarity of mind are acquired. While it is a fact that all sentient beings have Buddha nature, Buddhahood as such is only for the few; ordinary mortals must struggle on. For the great majority it is a matter rather of at least some alleviation of the human state. The late Toby Christmas-Humphreys never ceased to emphasize with repetitive monotony that in the final analysis – we are on our own. 'Walk On' was his constant and not always comforting admonition. How fortunate we are to have not only precious human bodies, but also gurus and spiritual companions to help and accompany us, on our quest for spiritual enlightenment. Providing we are willing to take the ultimate. responsibility the spiritually aware physician, whether Buddhist, Christian, Sufi or non-denominational, can help us achieve better health and happiness and at least relative freedom from disease and mental/emotional distress. This book just happens to be principally about the Buddhist and particularly the Tibetan approach in this respect.

The Wheel of Life

The Wheel[12] graphically depicts the whole of samsara (phenomenal existence) not only in terms of karma and rebirth in the long term but also the states of mental confusion as they occur *now*, and indeed continuously in this present life. The Three Poisons etc. are depicted at the hub. Then like spokes in a wheel there are six sections symbolizing the Six Realms.

The Three Higher Realms are the:

1. Human Realm;	based on pride and allied to passion.
2. God Realm; (Devas)	self-satisfaction and hedonism predominate, grasping is still operative.
3. Jealous Gods; (Asuras)	always quarrelling, envy dominates leading to fighting, intrigue, worry, anxiety.

The Three Lower Realms are the:

4. Animal Realm;	stupidity characterizes this realm. Applied to human life – a state of being unevolved, small minded and narrow, unimaginative, unable to adapt, reflex-thinking, smug and self-satisfied.

5. Hungry-Ghost Realm; (Pretas)	visualized as having big bellies and tiny mouths, can never get enough. They are miserly, greedy and never satisfied, having got things find they don't want them.
6. Hell Realms; (Avicci) two in number	based on anger and aggression (a) Hot hell — characterized by explosive anger with hot passion, (b) Cold hell — hidden cold anger, plus pride, sulking and withdrawal, resentful depression.

The Six Realms make up samsara — we are constantly in one or the other, throughout each life and as our consciousness passes on from this life to the next life.

The rim of the Wheel represents the twelve Nidanas, 'the twelvefold chain of causality whereby beings are ensnared life after life' (Blofeld). Yama the Lord of Death grasps the Wheel, and Sakyamuni Buddha is depicted pointing at the Wheel of the Dharma — the Buddhist alternative to a life of suffering, frustration and unsatisfactoriness (dukkha).

The Bardo or Intermediate State

There are a number of Bardos but here we are concerned principally with rebirth–life–death, which until Enlightenment is achieved is a continuous processing of building-up (anabolism) and dissolution (catabolism) of the Five Elements.

Rebirth

The process of rebirth is described in detail in the *Sutra of the Teaching of Nanda on Entry to the Womb*, quote: 'In the sixth to tenth months, the four elements, earth, water, fire and wind — and the space constituent are produced in the sense that their capacities reach fulfilment' (Lati Rinbochay).[13]

Life

Exemplified by metabolism, this is a continuous interplay of anabolism and catabolism (life and death in a momentary sense) with a split-second bardo state in between, until death.

Death

There are three phases in the process of dying normally:

1. The senses gradually fail;
2. The Five Elements dissolve;
3. Psychic awareness develops of the beyond physical death state and there is perception of the Clear Light outside of dimension, time and space.

The Five Elements dissolve in this order:

(a) Earth into Water;
(b) Water into Fire;
(c) Fire into Air;
(d) Air into Ineffable Awareness.

Mantras

John Blofeld[14] calls mantras — sacred words of power. Mantras express the archetypal sounds and energies essential to a harmonized balance of the Five Elements, the basic stuff of the universe, and consequently to the Three Humours in relation to the psychic channels and cakras. Bijas are one-syllable mantras, Dharanis are strings of Bijas. All are based on the basic articulated sounds of the Sanskrit alphabet. Lawrence Blair[15] describes a 'tonoscope', an instrument which transforms sounds uttered into a microphone into their visual representation on a screen. He says:

> The sacred Hindu syllable — OM, when correctly uttered into the tonoscope, apparently produces the circle 'O', which is then filled in with concentric squares and triangles, finally

producing, when the last traces of 'M' have died away, a 'yantra', the formal geometrical expression of sacred vibration, which is found in many of the world's religions.
(And particularly in Tantric Buddhism – T.G.D.)

The Bodhisattva

The Bodhisattva ideal belongs essentially and historically to the Indian Mahayana tradition of Buddhism, which eventually spread to Tibet and Mongolia in the ninth century AD to become the Vajrayana, and also to China to become Ch'an and to Japan to become Zen. Theravadin, or the basic Buddhism of Sri Lanka and South East Asia places emphasis on the achievement of Enlightenment by individuals as individuals in terms of the ultimate state of Nirvana, this being understood as being the opposite to Samsara – the world of everyday life and living. Those who are able to reach this exalted state are known as Arahants.

Bodhisattvas are 'enlightened-mind persons', who at some point in endless time, often as very ordinary and spiritually unevolved beings have nevertheless taken the Bodhisattva-vow. This is a firm commitment to follow the Bodhisattva path starting at the level of the 1st bhumi (see page 9) and of course is not taken lightly and always with the advice and consent of the spiritual Teacher.

In Tibetan the Bodhisattva-vow is as follows:

Chang chup sem ni rinpoche
Maje panam je jur chik
Je pa nyampa me pa tang
Gong ne Gong du pewar sho

This is literally translated as:

The Precious Bodhicitta,
Not arisen may it arise;
Having arisen, may it go
from height to height

Colloquially translated as:

> May I arouse Bodhicitta for the welfare
> of all sentient beings
> And may it develop in power, strength
> and activity without limit.

In practice taking the Bodhisattva-vow means putting oneself last, by foregoing personal Enlightenment in the Theravadin sense until all other sentient beings have achieved the same exalted state, and dedicating all one's efforts to helping towards this end.

Taking the Bodhisattva-vow means also practising the Six Paramitas as well as developing the Four Qualities for attracting beings who wish to be helped: giving, gentle speech, practice according to the meaning of the Dharma and encouraging others to act according to the meaning.

The Six Paramitas (or Transcending Perfections)

One day, in discussion with my Teacher, the Ven. Ato Rinpoche, I raised the subject of Tibetan medicine and healing generally. Without a moment's hesitation his advice shot back, direct and to the point – it all depends on attitude of mind. 'MIND-AWARENESS and the SIX PARAMITAS', said Rinpoche, 'constitute the fundamental basis for practising Tibetan Medicine.'

Mind-Awareness is the same as the Wisdom Mind mentioned above. It connotes the mind remaining in essential meditational equipoise devoid of conceptuality, thought or expression. This does not mean that the mind is necessarily still or always empty. It should be constructively occupied in a one-pointed, purposeful and disciplined way and in perfect rest between times.

The Six Paramitas are as follows:

1. the perfection of giving   – Dana Paramita;
2. the perfection of morality   – Sila Paramita;
3. the perfection of patience   – Ksanti Paramita;
4. the perfection of energy   – Virya Paramita;
5. the perfection of meditation– Dhyana Paramita;
6. the perfection of wisdom   – Prajna Paramita.

Table 3 The Eightfold Consciousness according to Mahayana Buddhism[16]

(A) Regarded as three layered	
1. Alaya Vijnana	(store consciousness)
2. Manas	(thought centre)
	(self-conscious mind)
3. Caksur Vijnana	(eye consciousness)
Srotra Vijnana	(ear consciousness)
Ghrana Vijnana	(nose consciousness)
Jihva Vijnana	(tongue consciousness)
Kaya Vijnana	(body or touch consciousness)
Mano Vijnana	(mind consciousness)

(B) Regarded as two layered	
1. Alaya Vijnana	(store consciousness)
2. Pravrttivijnanas	(evolved consciousness)
Manas	
Caksur Vijnana	
Srotra Vijnana	Darsanabhaga (perception)
Ghrana Vijnana	Nimittabhaga (image)
Jihva Vijnana	
Kaya Vijnana	
Mano Vijnana	

There are many levels of Teachings and indeed interpretations of the paramitas relevant to all the different life-aspects and activities.

Applied to medicine, giving and morality relate very much to the simple fact of always putting the patient first, to always be available whenever humanly possible, being there to help in whatever way is in the best interest of the patient, i.e. ethical discipline, even though what one advises or does may not always be what the patient wants or thinks is best, and by using upaya or skilful means in order to help. Acting in perfect empathy or practising maitri (active love in a detached, non-sentimental way) and giving Dharma advice wherever appropriate, but without as the Ven. Trungpa Rinpoche has said – 'invading the other person's territory', or even more colloquially – not laying one's own trip on the patient.

Patience in the presence of suffering is, perhaps, one of the most difficult perfections to practise in the consulting-room. It certainly needs energy which protects against tiredness to sustain it, i.e. diligence.

Meditation is the sure and certain way of developing and sustaining paramitas 1–4 and ultimately achieving Mind-Awareness, the certain key to tuning in to the ultimate essence of the Five-Elements level mentioned earlier on.

3

The Tibetan Medical Philosophy of Health

The subject matter of Tibetan medicine has been set out in an orderly and logical fashion in a manner very appealing to the Western mind by Dr Yeshi Donden and the Ven. Lobsang Rapgay, under the headings below.

(a) Tibetan Medical Philosophy
(b) The Healthy Body
(c) Humours
(d) The Seven Physical Energies
(e) Excretions
(f) The Unhealthy Body:
    (i) Functional Disorders
    (ii) Pathology
(g) Methods of Diagnosis
(h) Treatment by:
    (i) Diet
    (ii) Behavioural Therapy
    (iii) Medication
    (iv) Accessory Therapy

In the rGyud bZhi these are all traditionally described and discussed using the analogy of the Tree of Life, with its roots, branches and leaves – a perfect example of holism. The translation of this traditional arrangement of material has been meticulously reproduced in Dr Elisabeth Finckh's book *Foundations of Tibetan Medicine*, vol. 1. There is therefore no point in duplicating what has already been so admirably done.

Since, however, this particular book is primarily concerned with relating Tibetan medicine to other holistic systems and therapies and particularly in a Western context, the relevant and obviously condensed material is presented rather in terms of the format presented by Dr Yeshi Donden and the Ven. Lobsang Rapgay.[1]

In the previous two chapters the Buddhist foundations of the Tibetan medical system have been discussed at a depth which is hopefully adequate for the aspiring Western student. Buddhist literature in the English language alone is now so vast, certainly sufficient for a litetime's study, or a more superficial acquaintance, as one may wish.

Before passing on to the more specific aspects of Tibetan medical philosophy I can do no better than quote Dr Yeshi Donden and Mr Gyatso Tshering (Director of the Library of Tibetan Works and Archives, at Dharamsala):

The primary aim of Tibetan medicine as with all other systems of medicine is to relieve human beings of physical suffering, viz – to restore to equilibrium in this instance, imbalances in the normal functioning of the wind, bile and phlegm elements in the body that is the humours. It is true that one's mental disposition influences and determines, to a vast degree, the body functions, stresses and strains, and all other activities associated with the body. Mind is superior to body. Mind is the architect of all our sufferings and happiness. Mind is the master; body and speech are its attendants. While the cultivation of the art and science of medicine is predominantly intended to cure the physical ailments of a being, Tibetan physicians place an equal degree of stress on the cultivation and development of mental power and the observance of moral laws. For us Tibetans, the psychology, ethics and philosophy of Buddhism have provided abundant and effective means for controlling consciousness and preventing it from becoming wild or disarrayed. For the elimination of body suffering, the healing art of medicine is prescribed. For the modification of consciousness (mind), Dharma i.e. moral laws are prescribed. The two are closely related. Psychology, parapsychology, ethics and philosophy, as enunciated in the Dharma, are all conducive to and directed towards the controlling of the consciousness in order to obtain mental and bodily peace.... Tibetan medicine, firmly rooted in religion and philosophy, takes man as if a whole, in the empirical and transcendental aspects, as a physical entity and metaphysical potentiality. As a body, man is a microcosmic but faithful reflection of the macrocosmic reality in which he is imbedded and which preserves and nourishes him every second of his life; as a mind, he is a ripple on the surface of the great ocean of consciousness. Health is the proper relationship between the microcosm which is man and the macrocosm which is the Universe. Disease is a disruption of this relationship. Unimpeded reaction of the macrocosm to such a disruption results in a cure, unless the disruption is irreversible, when death becomes the cure. Certain elements, things and factors are of help in certain kinds of disease and become specifics for such diseases. The science of medicine is both descriptive and curative. The descriptive enumerates and describes the body and mind, their relationship, normal and abnormal functioning, their diseases, their symptoms and varieties, the remedial factors in nature-elements and minerals, plants and animals, and their preparation and combination.[2]

Tibetan medicine is thus seen to be truly cosmological and its philosophy and practice reflect accordingly in terms of the unity and interrelationship of all its various aspects.

The Five Cosmic Energies

Again, to quote Dr Yeshi Donden (and Lobsang Rapgay)

All animate and inanimate phenomena, according to Buddhism, have the same material basis, that is everything is composed of, or exists dependent upon the five cosmic energies. The five cosmic energies are simply translated earth, water, fire, air and space. The English equivalents, however, do not convey the real meaning of the terms. For example, ordinary water does not just contain water cosmic energy, rather it is composed of all cosmic energies.

It is on the theory of five cosmic energies that the sciences of anatomy, pathology and pharmacology are established. This means that when a person is suffering from a disorder, the disorder and the medication both have basically the same material composition. It was in reliance upon this theory that a physician would use his experience and knowledge in treating a patient. Using the law of similarity and dissimilarity accordingly, he would generally treat cold disorders with hot remedies and hot disorders with cold remedies.

As Jigme Tsarong says, 'The five cosmophysical energies are not static physio-chemical elements, but dynamic forces which deal more with the inherent energetical functions rather than their actual state'.

sa	Earth	: is involved in the formation of bones, muscles, skin and eyes, and for the sense of smell.
chu	Water	: is responsible for the formation of the body fluids — blood, lymph, etc., and also for the sense of taste.
me	Fire	: activates body temperature, is responsible for skin tone and a healthy complexion and the sense of sight.
rlung	Air	: the function of respiration and the sense of touch belongs to this element.
nam-mkh'a	Space	: the orifices and cavities of the body belong to space, as does the sense of hearing.

Relation of the Five Elements with the senses

sa	Earth	— smell
chu	Water	— taste
me	Fire	— sight
rlung	Air	— touch
nam-mkh'a	Space	— hearing

The Basic Causes of all Disease

The Five Elements in the body relate to the Five Elements in the environment, and medicines are also composed of the Four

Elements – Earth, Water, Fire and Air. When the elements are not balanced disease occurs (Dr Tenzin Choedak). This is in effect an expression of the 'Byung-ba lNga Theory which 'states that all physical phenomena, whether in the macrocosmic or micro-cosmic world, are formed by the five cosmo-physical energies' (four elements) (Jigme Tsarong).

The Buddhist belief and teaching concerning the basic causes of all disease starts at the primordial level with the Dug-gsum theory. Again I quote Jigme Tsarong who has worded it perfectly:

> Buddhism starts with the premise that everything within the universe is in a constant state of flux: that all phenomena are characterised by impermanence and that the only permanent feature is its impermanence. 'No matter whether perfect beings arise or not' the Buddha said 'it remains a fact and hard necessity of existence that all creation is transitory'.

It is this very impermanence of creation that causes each and every being, at one stage or another, to suffer. Suffering is not accidental but springs from a specific cause. The extinction of suffering means the liberation from the vicious cycle of existence, and this is accomplished through the proper knowledge and genuine practice of the Dharma.

The Three Poisons

'The Buddha traced the specific cause of all suffering to the concept of bdag-'dzin or ego which is manifested in the form of ma-rig-pa (ignorance). This in turn gives rise to 'dod-chags (attachment), zhe-sdang (hatred) and gti-mug (closed-mindedness).

In comparing these Three Poisons with a fire which perma-nently consumed humanity, the Buddha said: "It burns through the fire of delusion, through the fire of attachment, through the fire of hatred: it burns through birth, old age and death; through grief, lamentation, pain, sorrow and despair."

The Three Poisons of 'dod-chags, zhe-sdang and gti-mug,

respectively, give rise to the three afflictions of rlung, mkhris-pa and bad-kan.*

An in-depth study of the Three Poisons is found in Buddhist philosophy and psychology and for our purpose it is important to note the close interrelationship between a mental and a physical disorder.'

As will be seen in Chapter 4, the etiology of disease is not found on the primordial level only. Various elements and influences are operative in our daily lives, and improper diet and harmful behavioural patterns, for instance, can upset the homeostatic equilibrium and operate as immediate causes.

Jigme Tsarong[3] gives a definition of the art of healing in the context of Tibetan Medicine as follows:

> The whole art of healing in this tradition, involves the proper aligning of the three divisions, in a dynamic state of equilibrium and homeostasis.

The Body in its Natural Condition of Health

With and beyond the visible man there is a vast area of invisible forces, currents and vibratory structures, inaccessible to the senses, but nevertheless entirely real, concrete. They are essential for the proper functioning of the body and mind, and constitute the subtle counterpart of the gross physical body. They may be described as Bile, Air and Phlegm – the three Humours.

As Theodore Burang says:

> The meaning of 'bile' in Tibetan humoral pathology is not the substance known to us as bile, but the subtle principle which is its equivalent. The same applies to 'air' and 'phlegm'. . . .
> According to ancient Indian medical philosophy, upon which Tibetan healers have largely drawn, 'air', 'bile' and 'phlegm' correspond to the principles of mind, energy and inert matter. . . . The dominant characteristics of the three humours

---

* rLung – loong = Wind
  mKhris-pa – tripa – tipa = Bile
  bad-kan – peh-ken = Phlegm

are as follows: air is light and dry, bile is hot, phlegm is cold, viscous and heavy.[4]

Theodore Burang[5] on page 25 of his book, describes the life-force cycle, which circulates in opposite directions in the male and female. The nadis and chakras and the three largest channels through which these subtle principles flow are called 'ro-ma', 'u-ma'* and 'rkyang-ma', and are said to wind themselves in a corkscrew fashion around the spinal column. The spinal column is considered to be the axial centre of the Universe – the mythical Mount Meru, the abode of the gods. These channels are often referred to as 'veins', but again are not to be confused with the normal, physical blood vessels, i.e. solely in a Western sense. However, as previously mentioned, Keith Dowman points out – 'The word for psychic nerves (rtsa, nadi) is the same as for the veins and arteries, and for tendons and muscles'.[6] The implication here is – 'a parallel in the body's physiology and also in the mental sphere, for the subtle, the gross and the mental inter-relate', i.e. in Tantric Buddhist thinking. Also in Tantric literature the word bindu (or thig-le) frequently appears. Traditionally this refers to 'seed-essence'. Herrick designates this as 'creative-potentiality'. On the physical level this is semen.

The Three Humours

To re-state – the Three Humours are:

Wind   – (rLung)
Bile   – (mKhris-pa)
Phlegm – (Bad-kan)

These are divided into:

Five basic Winds
Five basic Biles
Five basic Phlegms

* in Tibetan spelled dbu-ma

The five psychocosmic energies or elements referred to above relate to the Three Humours as follows:

Air   – rLung
Fire   – mKhris-pa
Earth and Water – Bad-kan

The five different types of Humour are:

Bile	*Air*	*Phlegm*
1. Digestive – generates body heat and digests food and facilitates proper function of the other 'Biles'	Life–Wind – holds the Life-force; gives a special clarity to the mind and binds mind and body together	Mixing and Decomposing – mixes bolus together and decomposes it
2. Colour regulating – controls and regulates pigmentation, colour of blood, nutriment, etc.	Upward moving – gives clarity of mindfulness, associated with bodily strength and colour and gives energy	Experiencing and Tasting – facilitates gustatory functions (experiencing tastes)
3. Sense of Achievement – contributes to pride, intelligence, realizing desires and self-confidence	Pervasive – flows through whole body – concerned with movement of limbs, thinking processes, regulates blood circulation – opening and closing of apertures	Connecting – synchronizes joint-function and muscular contraction and relaxation
4. Visual ability – facilitates vision and appreciation of form	Fire associated – moves through all hollow organs, separates nutritives from waste and facilitates absorption	Satisfying – responsible for sense-organ satisfaction
5. Complexion-clearing – gives a clear skin and regulates its colour	Downward voiding – concerned with pelvic secretory organs and thighs	Supporting – regulates peristalsis in the oesophagus, provides lubrication (mucus, etc.)

Centres or locations of the different Humours:

Bile	Air	Phlegm
1. 2nd and 3rd Levels of the Stomach	Crown of the Head	Lower Oesophagus
2. Liver	Centre of the Chest	Tongue
3. Heart	Heart	Joints
4. Eyes	3rd Level of the Stomach	Top of Head
5. Skin	Lower Abdomen	Lower Chest along Breast Bone

The Seven Basic Body Constituents

In addition there are the seven basic body constituents:

1. the nutritive qualities of the food (essence) – Dangs-ma
2. Blood – Khrag
3. Flesh – Sha
4. Fat (including gristle) – Tsil
5. Bone – Rus
6. Bone-marrow – rKang
7. the regenerative fluids Semen and Ovum[7] – Khu-ba

Dangs-ma forms khrag, khrag forms sha, sha forms tsil, tsil forms rus, rus forms rkang and rkang forms khu-ba.

In addition there are the three excretory substances:

(a) Bowel excreta
(b) Urine
(c) Perspiration or sweat.

In order to maintain homeostasis these different aspects, functions and energies must be in dynamic functional relationship both individually and in groups (systems) with each other and in terms of the whole – body, speech and mind. The balance between the fifteen Humours and the ten different aspects, functions and energies = Good Health.

Notes on the Seven Basic Body Constituents

1. *Nutrition* The nutritive qualities of food – this is the pure essence of digested food. Since the body is formed (and kept in health) by this essence, it is most important that absorption should be 100 per cent.
2. *Blood* Supports life, is essential to all life-processes, and maintains communication between structure and function (the body and its activities).
3. *Flesh* Represents growth and the formation of the body and covers the body.
4. *Fat (and gristle)* Maintains body tonus and lubricates.
5. *Bones* The solid foundation of the body.
6. *Bone-Marrow* Fortifies and is essential for body-strength.
7. *Reproductive Liquids* Facilitate reproduction and new life.

Excretions

The Three Excretory Substances and Functions

1. *Bowels and defaecation*: excess – diarrhoea
   insufficient – constipation
   (this is often a rLung or Wind problem)
2. *Urine and micturition*: urine deficient – body colour is lost.
3. *Skin and perspiration*: (i) normal – good skin function
   (ii) excess will cause skin ailments
   (iii) insufficient – the skin cracks and peels or flakes off.

Environmental Influence

Concerning the environment the five cosmo-physical energies or elements influence the body through the humours as follows:

Air – wind, turbulence or airlessness, affecting Wind (humour).
Fire – heat affecting Bile.
Earth and Water – dampness and humidity affecting Phlegm.

Conception and Embryology

A detailed account in Chapter 2 of the Explanatory Tantra is given on the development and growth of the foetus in utero (Ambrosia Heart Tantra). Dr Tenzin Choedak is adamant that the mother should observe a proper diet and behavioural pattern during pregnancy otherwise the child may be deformed. Contact with chemicals in any shape or form is particularly harmful. Also parents must be healthy otherwise conception may not take place. An excess of the Bile humour, he says, may also prevent conception.

The bShad rgyud* says that concerning conception itself the uterus is only ready to conceive during the twelve days after menstruation is finished; it is said that during that period 'the lotus is fully open'. The bShad rgyud* also says – 'Like the closing of the lotus after sunset, once twelve days have passed (after the end of the menstrual period) the womb does not receive semen'.

Three factors are necessary – *sperm*, *ovum* and *consciousness* meeting, the result having the appearance of curd that is pure white in colour. The whiteness is associated with the Wind humour. If the Bile humour is in excess the whiteness will be replaced by a yellowish appearance, and with an excess of the Phlegm humour the substance will become lumpy (Dr Tenzin Choedak).

The text also goes into some detail concerning sex determination, for example:

(a) a preponderance of sperm over ovum favours a male child;
(b) the reverse favours a female child;
(c) an equal amount of both sperm and ovum may result in twins being conceived.

During confinement it is said that if the foetus in utero moves to the right side of the mother's abdomen the child will be male, and vice versa. Moreover if the right breast of the mother appears

---

* Explanatory Tantra

larger the child will be male and if the left breast is bigger — a female.[9]

In the commentary to the Kalacakra Tantra His Holiness the Dalai Lama states:

> In ordinary rebirth, a being in the intermediate state between the last life and the new life sees its father and mother lying together. If the being is to be reborn as a male, he desires the mother and wants to separate from (get rid of) the father. If the being is to be reborn as a female, she desires the father and wants to separate from (get rid of) the mother. When the being, out of wanting to copulate, begins to embrace the one that is desired, he or she perceives only the partner's sexual organ, due to which he/she becomes frustrated and angry. In the midst of desire and anger, the being of the intermediate state dies and thereupon enters the womb, and is reborn in the sense that conception takes place.[10]

The Six Tastes

The qualities and energy-functions of the five cosmo-physical energies will be discussed in Chapter 9, which deals with the materia medica and medication therapy. Basically, these consist of six combinations in pairs of the four elements — for example, Earth, Water, Fire and Air produce the Six Tastes: sweet, sour, salty, bitter, acrid and astringent, qualities which belong to both foods and medicines.

Thus, unsuitable items of food or drink may upset the balance of the three Humours. Further to this they will exert either an aggravating or ameliorating influence, either singly or in combination, on disorders of the humours. Therapeutically the properties of the Six Tastes are applied selectively in a pharmacodynamic sense as 'alteratives' (see *Fundamentals of Tibetan Medicine*, pp. 32–8).

Conscious Expansion

In conclusion, in his essay on 'Conscious Expansion'[11] Lama Govinda epitomizes pertinent to Tibetan medical philosophy, the

cosmological relationships between *homo sapiens*, the microcosm, and the boundless environment, the macrocosm, particularly in terms of the inner silent point within us all (for the
finding) which in Buddhist terms is the centre of the
Tathagatagarba or 'Buddha-nature'. He writes:

> The mere 'expansion' of consciousness has no value unless we
> have found our inner centre* in which all the faculties of mind
> and psyche are integrated and to which all our experiences are
> referred as their ultimate judge and arbiter. This inner centre is
> situated between the poles of the individual peripheric
> consciousness of the intellect and the non-individual depth-
> consciousness in which we partake of the greater life of the
> universe. When this centre functions rightly the whole
> impression is one of evident harmony with inner life. The inner
> and the outer exist not against but for each other.
>
> Always then the presence of the basic vital centre is
> expressed in the easy equilibrium of the two poles and if one
> preponderates over the other the result is a wrong relation to
> heaven and earth, to the world and to the self.
>
> Just as failure to achieve the right centre always implies a
> disturbance of the living whole so the achievement of it
> demonstrates nothing less than that state in which the *whole* is
> kept alive *in the right tension between the two poles*.
>
> The tendency towards centralisation is not only a biological
> and psychological necessity, but a law of universal dynamics,
> pervading the entire cosmos – irrespective whether applied to
> spiral nebulae or solar systems, planets or electrons. Every
> movement has a tendency to create its own centre or its own
> axis, as the only possible form of stability within the infinite
> movement of all that lives.
>
> Where, however, life becomes conscious of itself, there a
> new, subtler centralisation takes place in a consciousness that
> creates its own focus, moving as if it were on a infinite axis
> from distant past towards an equally distant future (as it

---

* Professor Laborit has in a Western scientific context explained how human
reactions in a physio-chemical sense also oscillate around a 'fixed-point' – see
Chapter 11.

appears to us), or more correctly: which moves towards a present that (to us) is in a state of continual transformation.

Western Observations

Furthermore, a primary Western researcher into Tibetan medicine, Elisabeth Finckh, sums up very succinctly the whole matter of studying and hopefully understanding Tibetan medicine:

> Tibetan medicine is a holistic therapy. The system of Tibetan medicine almost always depends upon this three-part division; diagnosis and therapy are held to be impossible without knowledge of the three humours, and this is borne out in practice. Tibetan medicine is above all a doctrine of constitution. The concept that the body with its anatomical, physiological, psychic and intellectual functions acts as a mirror of the macrocosm should be mentioned as a further important aspect. This world of analogies, of corresponding phenomena, in which fine sub-strata of a non-material nature make possible an inter-reaction of body and mind cannot be compared with our Western concepts and can hardly be explained in Western terms. We can merely observe that Tibetan medicine is primarily orientated towards functions and not towards material sub-strata.[12]

The 'Flowers' and 'Fruits' of Health

The logical sequence of the body in its natural condition of health results in:

1. Two Flowers, and
2. Three Fruits.

The first Flower is freedom from disease and the *second Flower* is long-life.
The first Fruit is Dharma:

(a) Worldly Dharma; i.e. the development of good (noble) human characteristics, and

(b) Divine Dharma; the following of a particular religious path.

The second Fruit is wealth:

(a) Material wealth, and
(b) Spiritual wealth in terms of the seven aryan possessions, having:
1. a pure teacher (guru) and the capacity to follow him;
2. ethics and generosity;
3. the capacity to apply the Teachings of the Dharma in one's own mind;
4. a sense of appropriate action (social consciousness);
5. the necessary sensitivity in order to avoid negative actions;
6. the ability to be ashamed of oneself if having indulged in negative behaviour, i.e. so that positive karma results instead;
7. the sensitivity to understand the Dharma.

The third Fruit is happiness, having the capacity:

(a) to pass one's own life in a state of happiness and being able to create happiness around oneself, and
(b) to free oneself from confusion and ignorance and attain liberation (Enlightenment).

Conclusion

In conclusion it may be said that there are two branches or aspects of Tibetan medicine:

(a) the 'Fundamental' (holistic and spiritual) based on Dharma is therefore basic Buddhist medicine. This involves not only a clinical assessment on the 'gross body', i.e. material level, but an evaluation of the patient's health problem on the 'subtle body' if not the 'very subtle body' level. Pulse diagnosis is a basic tool through which the deepest causes (spiritual) of humoural imbalance are evaluated.[13]

(b) the 'Symptomatic' approach as exemplified in the 3rd Tantra is based more on Ayurvedic and Chinese medicine principles, where the spiritual basis is perhaps less evident than in Tibetan medicine. This more material basis reflects rather a Vade Mecum approach of specific treatments for specific diseases. Pulse diagnosis, although it is invariably used by Tibetan doctors as a stratagem in order to relate and empathize with the patient, does not have any fundamental diagnostic purpose other than that (please refer to Chapter 8).[14]

4

Disease

The unhealthy body basically reflects imbalanced functioning of the fifteen humours, the seven physical energies and the three excretions.

Etiology

The causes of disease are distant and/or immediate. They are equally multiple, excepting for the fundamental first cause mentioned in the previous chapter,* i.e. what is sometimes called 'the universal long-term cause of disease' which is ignorance* or (marigpa) and as explained in that context, then gives rise to 'dod-chags, zhe-sdang and ti-mug. By the same token the Three Mental Poisons are the originating causes of the Three Humours themselves, and at that point are still obviously long-term causes. Immediate causes of disease are found in the imbalances between the Three Humours, the seven physical energies and the three excretory functions themselves.

Etiologically there are four principal groups of causes:

(a) By negative actions in former lives (karma – cause and effect).

(b) Those which operate again on a karmic cause and effect

* Ignorance is the root cause of all diseases – ignorance of how the self really exists. It causes rebirth into cyclic existence (the Twelve Nidanas – the Wheel of Life) resulting in suffering, disease, old age and death.

basis as a result of negative actions in this life but at an earlier period.

(c) Disturbing factors that often, but not always, make their presence felt later in life: incompatible behaviour, excesses and abuses, unsuitable diet, seasonal and occasional influences, trauma including injury by weapons, stress, deprivation, environmental and ecological reasons.

(d) 'Possession' by spirit entities – nagas, demons. Traditionally, diseases caused by evil spirits come next in importance after karmic diseases. Perhaps from a Western point of view we would be inclined to put them last as being of no consequence?

It is interesting that within this context Tibetan medicine postulates the possibility of what Western medicine understands by infection by micro-organism. For example viruses would seem to approximate with demons (Klu). This is a subject however which is never clearly explained, at least that has been my experience to date.

While on the subject of 'possession', I well remember a clinical incident when in Dharamsala, India, in 1977. One day I was with Lama Yeshe Dorje Rinpoche, a Ngag-pa, that is a yogi possessed of magical and healing powers, an exorcist and rain-maker, who is particularly adept in divination and ritual medicine. A young Indian lad had come to consult him regarding an intractable skin problem affecting a hand. Running sores are not uncommon in this environment and are often due to no more than malnutrition and/or infection. The young man gave no impression of being under-nourished and had been attending both the Tibetan Medical Centre, and later the Dharamsala Hospital where he had been treated by antibiotics and steroid ointments, with some improvement but no cure as such. Rinpoche was quite specific and to the point – the hand would not clear up because there was a naga (snake demon) lodged inside and only ritual means would deal with it. I was unable to follow up on this particular case as I left Dharamsala shortly afterwards, but I do know that this sort of clinical problem is a daily happening in Rinpoche's present life. Incidentally Rinpoche has been recognized as a 'very high Being' by the Great 5th Dalai Lama, and his lineage as a Tulku (reincarnate Lama) dates from that period.

After this strange digression – strange perhaps to our Western culture – let us return to a discussion of the immediate causes of disease:

1. Incompatible behaviour.
2. Diet as a causative factor.
3. The influence of age and biotypological factors on the humours.
4. Daily, seasonal and geographical influences.
5. The three circumstances relative to diseases arising.

As Dr Trogawa Rinpoche says – in establishing the etiology or cause of disease, all influences: behavioural patterns, diet, seasonal factors (time of year) and particularly the 'Imbalance of the Seasons' and decade of life must be taken into consideration.[1]

1.   Incompatible Behaviour

This concerns body, speech and mind and the harmful effects of extremes of behaviour. Over-activity is just as harmful as under-activity on all three levels. For example, taking the body aspect first, idleness expresses itself in two ways:

(a) an actual lack of physical activity or
(b) the frustration occasioned by not being able to indulge in an activity that one would like to do.

Physical exercise, whether it be work, sport or gymnastics, can actually be traumatizing in itself and is likely to be equally harmful. As with the effects of actual trauma this is particularly so on an empty stomach. Breath-holding is also very potentially harmful.

The dangers of idleness or overdoing it apply equally to activities involving speech and mind. Body and speech are like servants, they are controlled by the mind, so it is imperative that the mind be neither over nor under-active.

Occasional Behaviour as a Factor

Chapter 15 of the *Explanatory Tantra* is specific in its advice –

> Do not obstruct the impulses of hunger, thirst, vomiting, yawning, sneezing, breathing, sleeping, to clear mucus from the throat, to remove excess saliva from the mouth and throat. Do not suppress the desire to defaecate or urinate, do not hold or suppress intestinal wind and gas or block the emission of semen. . . . By obstructing (or alternatively forcing these actions), all ailments arise and the winds are immediately disturbed.

Wind

This is one of the basic causes of *all* disease. Energy is disturbed by too much mental pressure, sadness, talkativeness, crying and sex. Also insufficient sleep or food, heavy intake of stimulants, eating 'foodless foods' (junkfood), fasting and extreme dieting, giving too much blood (blood donors beware), haemorrhage, excessive vomiting and diarrhoea, exhaustion from excessive sexual intercourse, sitting in a cold draught or wind. Stress is the over-riding factor. By causing mind disturbances the Wind in the body is disturbed. It is not surprising that Wind disturbances are much more common in the West. They were almost non-existent in Tibet before the Chinese invasion and occupation.

Bile

Hatred towards others and anger are the main causes of Bile problems. Too much sun-bathing and excessive exercise and sport are conducive to Bile upsets.

Phlegm

Big meals and particularly sleeping afterwards (including relaxing after meals), contact with cold water, cold and damp places. Sleeping during the day and swimming during spring and winter also favour Phlegm disturbances.

The Relevance of the Three Humours

(a) Wind+ generally perturbs
Bile+ overheats
Phlegm+ blocks and obstructs due to its heavy and sticky nature.

(b) Wind is aggravated by cold
Bile is aggravated by heat
Phlegm is aggravated by damp (cold).[2]

2. Diet as a Causative Factor

Unsuitable diet, that is an imbalanced diet for the person concerned, can block the vital channels. When the smaller channels are blocked, this may only cause insidious and minor health problems. Since health depends on the latter being kept open and, equally, the blood vessels and excretory channels, a suitable diet means one that is balanced and moderate that also accords with the person's typology.

Basically, in health one should eat everything (a vindication of the time-honoured Western medical advice that the best diet is a mixed diet) but in moderation. Remember the old adage – 'one third of what we eat keeps us alive, the other two-thirds keeps doctors alive'. So as far as nutrition is concerned in health, it's moderation and balance that matters, and having found it one should not dwell on the matter any further. Another interpretation if you like of the old osteopathic precept of 'Find it – fix it and leave it alone'.

In disease one should regulate food intake according to the involvement or imbalance of the Three Humours and, where specifically indicated, eliminate for the time being relevant articles of diet that will only aggravate existing imbalances.

Wind disturbances and diseases can be caused or exacerbated by excesses of: pork, goat meat, strong tea and coffee, the flesh of wild animals and birds, vegetable oils (particularly those made from grains), unripe fruit and vegetables, sugar, cold drinks, cold foods. Also by bitter-tasting, coarse and light foods and water. Alcohol is normally all right in health, if taken in very strict moderation only.

Alimentary symptoms which indicate an excess of the Wind humour are: excessive hunger, voracious appetite, the person who eats big meals often at regular intervals, frequently suffers from indigestion and constipation (the latter is often an expression of Wind imbalance, and the former rather of Phlegm imbalance).

Rechung Rinpoche points out that when a person is about to contract a disease of air (Wind) foods harmful to diseases of air are craved, and there is no desire for those which are beneficial to air diseases.[3] It is also of interest that garlic and onions are good for balancing the Wind humour, but too much upsets the balance and can cause diseases other than those of Wind origin.

Bile disturbances and diseases can be caused or exacerbated by excesses of: red meat (beef and lamb), eggs, nut-butters and particularly peanut butter, brown sugar and onions. Also an excess of sharp, hot, sour and salty foods and beer and alcohol generally.

Alimentary signs of too much Bile are: generally the person seems to be able to eat a lot and digest well, but this is provided that the digestive capacity is not overloaded, otherwise gross or uncompensated imbalance will arise.

Too much rich food generally and particularly the foods mentioned in this category can cause 'blockage' or obstruction in the larger blood vessels and give rise to circulatory troubles and ultimately cancer. As Dr Tenzin Choedhak remarked, the problem is then obvious.

Phlegm disturbances and diseases can be caused or aggravated by excesses of: goat-meat, milk, tea, butter, yoghourt, fat, grain oils (including mustard), peanut and sunflower oil, fresh grains, raw fresh vegetables (raw foods generally), garlic and onions, unripe fruit. Too much cold, heavy, greasy, bitter and sweet food and left-overs of both food and drink, and over-eating generally.

Alimentary symptoms arising from too much phlegm are: the person has a small appetite, eats very little and frequently suffers from indigestion.

Dr Tenzin Choedhak[4] says that the medical texts lay great emphasis on the possible harmful chemical reactions brought about by wrong mixtures and combinations of food, for example:

chicken and yoghourt
eggs and fish

fish and milk	curd with new wine
peanuts and honey	milk with walnuts
honey and melted butter or oil	peaches with other fruit

T. Clifford gives the reason for this – 'Certain combinations of food are thought to be highly poisonous because each food is strongly influencing different humours, either negating the good qualities of each other, or having a combined effect that is deleterious'.[5]

In respect of potentially harmful food mixtures, T. Burang mentions – 'It should be remembered that the Central Asian sometimes reacts differently to the Westerner, even under the same external conditions'.[6]

Diet, the Humours and the Vital Channels

1. It is most important to give overriding attention to wind-energy disorders. Imbalances of Wind can cause involvement and imbalances of the other humours – Bile and Phlegm.
2. Excessive 'blockages' of the vital channels can cause bloatedness.
3. Wrong diet generally can block the vital channels.
4. Heat or warmth generally helps digestion – if a person is cold or their temperature decreases the digestive capacity is reduced. If there is insufficient heat in the stomach (the most important part of the body) the essence (essential nutriment) of the food will not be absorbed. A loss of stomach heat in the foetus for example could be due to the improper diet of the mother.

Digestive Fire

Digestive fire is like a machine; diets are the raw materials and bodily elements are the products. No one can expect a good product from a defective machine even if the raw materials are of very good quality. Similarly, weak digestion will serve the body with no healthy elements or tissues. For example, one can find a very weak and skinny son in a wealthy family which can afford the best foods available, while on the other hand, strong and healthy people can be found in poor families who live on very simple food. What is the reason for this contradiction? A person should have good digestion so that the food eaten will be assimilated by the body. It is said in the Tibetan medical texts that almost all of the chronic and internal diseases originate from indigestion. So it is very important to maintain the digestive fire. (Dr Pema Dorjee, TMI News-letter, June 1985)

Miscellaneous Observations[7]

(Dr Choedhak)

1. Sour foods and raw foods can block the vital channels and consequently imbalance the Humours and give rise to disease.
2. Meat, onions, garlic, salt and sugar and rich foods generally are contra-indicated in cancer, but not fish.
3. In obesity, qualitatively eat a good mixed diet but quantitatively *eat* less, he advises.

(Dr Trogawa Rinpoche)

1. Food intake must be adjusted to age and basic digestive capacity: With poor digestion – light and hot foods are advised and with 'heat+' type digestion – heavier but cooler foods are more suitable (too much heat in the stomach).
2. Poor diet may be a factor in disease, but it will be more actively etiologically if the time it is taken coincides with the moment in time that this or that disease would be most likely to arise seasonally.

3. The Influence of Age and Biotypological Factors on the Humours

There is a natural tendency for the humours to be relatively more active during the first three decades of life. This factor plus the individual biotypology* and tendencies of the person concerned

---

* The study of morphological differences between people. See Chapter 5, p. 82 and Appendix 1.

Table 4 Climatic and seasonal influences on the body and its disorders

The Tibetan year is divided into six seasons of two months each:		
Lower Winter	January/February	(11th & 12th months)
Spring	March/April	(1st & 2nd months)
Late Spring, Early Summer	May/June	(3rd & 4th months)
Summer (Monsoon)	July/August	(5th and 6th months)
Autumn	September/October	(7th & 8th months)
Upper Winter	November/December	(9th & 10th months)

are succinctly explained by T. Clifford:

> Bodily types and dispositions are also associated with the three humours. For example, babies have a great predominance of Phlegm. In the case of a baby that is a normal predominance for that life-stage, but in an adult, it would be a sickness due to Phlegm.[8]

Similarly, an adult person is dominated by Bile and an elderly person is dominated by Wind.

According to the Tibetan tradition:

(a) Childhood extends from 0–16 years;
(b) Adulthood and maturity extends from 16–70 years;
(c) Old age is 70 years onwards.

These calculations were made at the time of the Buddha when the average life-span was 100 years. Nowadays relative adjustment should be made (Barry Clark).

4. Daily, Seasonal and Geographical Influences

As T. Clifford also mentions: 'Astrology and the cycles of time* figure very importantly in Tibetan medicine; each humour is also

---

* Kalacakra Tantra.

Table 5 Relationship between disorders and seasonal changes

Tibetan month	Seasons	Accumulation	Rise	Decline
11 & 12	Lower Winter	Phlegm		
1 & 2	Spring		Phlegm	
3 & 4	Sos-ka	Wind		Phlegm
5 & 6	Summer (Monsoon)	Bile	Wind	
7 & 8	Autumn		Bile	Wind
9 & 10	Upper Winter			Bile

associated with a particular daily period, yearly season and a stage of life during which time it predominates'.[9]

(a) Daily Time Influences

1. The rising periods of Wind: evening and just before the dawn.
2. The rising periods of Bile: mid-day and midnight.
3. The rising periods of Phlegm: morning.

(b) The Seasonal Influence

The year is divided into six seasons:

1. The spring – months 1 and 2 of the Tibetan calendar.
2. Sos-ka, the first part of summer – months 3 and 4 of the Tibetan calendar.
3. The second half of summer – months 5 and 6 of the Tibetan calendar.
4. Autumn – months 7 and 8 of the Tibetan calendar.
5. The first part of winter – months 9 and 10 of the Tibetan calendar.
6. The second half of winter – months 11 and 12 of the Tibetan calendar.

No. 2, sos-ka, has a special significance being the hot and dry period. As Jigme Tsarong says:

> This is a period when the overall cosmo-physical energies are light and rough. This is also a period when Wind energies accumulate and can be further aggravated by light and rough dietary and behavioural regimes such as consuming too much garlic or excessive fasting. With the advent of summer and the heavy rains (monsoons) accompanied by strong and gusty winds, this gives rise to Wind energies. Thus the individual who has not paid proper attention to his diet and behaviour during sos-ka, will invariably suffer from a Wind disorder. The other two humours are similarly influenced by the seasons.[10]

Wind diseases:

  (i) accumulate at sos-ka;
 (ii) rise and manifest in the summer;
(iii) decline in the autumn.

Bile diseases:

  (i) accumulate in summer;
 (ii) rise and manifest in autumn;
(iii) decline in sos-ka the first part of winter.

Phlegm diseases:

  (i) accumulate during the second half of winter;
 (ii) rise and manifest in spring;
(iii) decline in sos-ka.

The Tibetan Year and Calendar

The Tibetan calendar is similar to the Chinese inasmuch as they divide the year into lunar months, designating them as the first, second months, etc. Generally every third year an extra month is inserted so as to make the calendar correspond with the solar years. Csoma de Koros says – 'The most common mode of reckoning time among people at large, especially in calculating the years of the present generation, or estimating the age of individuals, is that by the cycle of 12 years, in which each year is denominated from a certain animal... But in books, epistolary correspondence, and in every transaction of importance, the Tibetans made use generally of the cycle of 60 years. In 1986, we are at present in the Fire Tiger Year.'

The Tibetan pulse calendar has 360 days and is divided into twenty parts consisting of eighty days each of which relate to the six seasons and the Five Elements. As Jigme Tsarong says, 'It is imperative for the physician to know the exact season while checking the pulse or else his diagnosis may prove to be wrong.' Both RIGPA and Kham Tibetan House publish illustrated Tibetan calendars annually, in both the Tibetan and English languages.

Some Exceptions to Seasonal Aspects

Certain seasonal aspects described here do not necessarily apply in other parts of the world that are outside of the Himalayan, Central Asian countries and India. For example, the monsoon period is particular to those countries and areas. Also the six seasons are apparent in these parts of the world, whereas in Europe there are four distinct seasons. In Australia spring and autumn are very short, whereas summer and winter are longer depending on the area.

(c) Geographical Factors

    (i) Cold and windy places and climates favour the manifestation of Wind diseases.

   (ii) Hot and dry areas and climates encourage the appearance of Bile diseases.

  (iii) Damp places and climates aggravate and can give rise to Phlegm diseases.

There are three circumstances relative to diseases arising:

1. The starting-point, which involves a seasonal time-factor: for example the hot, cold and rainy seasons that are sos-ka, winter and summer proper.
2. The accumulation stage.
3. The actual manifestation of the disease.

It is very important to realize the relativity of all this. What is called the 'Imbalance of the Seasons' applies here. The hot season is not a fixed entity. It must be considered in relative terms of being more or less hot if, for example, during what is normally the hottest period of the hot season it happens to be much cooler than usual. The same applies equally for the cold season. The humours tend to be imbalanced accordingly.

Pathology

Pathological Entrance: the 'Doors of Disease' and Pathways of Disease

This process starts at the periphery with the skin and, considered in association with the various etiological factors already discussed, proceeds inwards, finally affecting the viscera. Dr Pema Dorje and Elizabeth Richards describe the process quite graphically:

> The 'Six Entrances' are the sites where disease manifests. In general, symptoms show in these places in the following order:
> Disease – scatters in the SKIN
> develops within the FLESH
> circulates in the CHANNELS
> holds to the BONES
> alights on the VITAL ORGANS
> and drops into any of the SIX VESSELS or HOLLOW ORGANS.[11]

The Five Vital Organs are

1. Heart
2. Liver

3. Lungs
4. Spleen
5. Kidneys

The Six Vessels or Hollow Organs are:

1. Stomach
2. Large intestine
3. Gall-bladder
4. Urinary bladder
5. Small intestine
6. Seminal vesicle or uterus*

According to the Root Tantra (the Basis of Illness) the general locations of the Three Humours are as follows:

Wind depends on the hipbones and the base of the spine and remains in the lower portion of the body.
Bile depends on the lining of the liver and remains in the middle portion of the body.
Phlegm depends upon the brain and remains in the upper portion of the body.

Dr Trogawa Rinpoche has elaborated interestingly in referring to the behaviour of a specific branch of Wind, Bile and Phlegm in each case, but not to general Wind, Bile and Phlegm. Examples of specific branches are as follows:

(a) *Wind* — hip–joints, peripheral joints, displaced Wind will 'lodge' in the lower extremities and large intestine.

(b) *Bile* — is mainly situated between the digested and undigested food in the stomach and 'lodges' in the throat and glottis.

(c) *Phlegm* — the main place of Phlegm is on top of the undigested food in the stomach. This is where

---

* Barry Clark remarks that Sam-se is commonly translated as 'nutriment vesicle', or 'ovaries' would be the most likely female equivalent — the translation is still under discussion and the exact meaning is still unresolved.

disease actually starts and then it moves elsewhere.

The Fifteen Directions or Movements of Disease

There are five directions of movements associated with three disturbed humours, making fifteen in all.

Wind — 1. Skin
2. Bones
3. Ears
4. Life-force vein in heart (vagus)
5. Large intestine.

Bile — 1. Blood
2. Sweat-glands
3. Eyes
4. Liver
5. Gall-bladder and small intestine.

Phlegm — 1. Muscle, fat, bone marrow and regenerative fluids
2. Nose and tongue
3. Urinary and defaecation passages
4. Lungs, spleen, kidneys
5. Stomach and urinary bladder.

The Classification of Illness

According to the *Explanatory Tantra* there are three basic classifications of illness with respect to:

1. The cause;
2. The type of patient;
3. The characteristics of the illness.

This may be elaborated in terms of:

1. The Cause

There are three classes of ailments that arise due to:

(a) disturbances of humours in this lifetime;
(b) from the karma (action) of previous lifetimes;
(c) a combination of (a) and (b).

There are three types relating to:

(a) (i) minor ailments;
    (ii) illnesses caused by spirits;
    (iii) some unwholesome action committed in the early stage of this present life.

with (b) those ailments due to karma (actions) of previous lifetimes rapidly worsen without any apparent reason.

  (c) illnesses due to a combination of the above (a and b) the patient often rapidly deteriorates due to a seemingly minor cause.

There are two further broad classifications of illness, those which arise due to:

(i) Internal causes, that is intrinsic, due to disturbances of the humours;
(ii) External causes, that is extrinsic, due to poisons, weapons (trauma) and demons, etc.

2.   The Ailments Affecting Different Types of Patients

These are five ailments of:

(a) Males
(b) Females
(c) Children
(d) Elderly people
(e) General ailments common to everyone.

The text then goes on to list in detail the various conditions pertaining to each type of patient: male, female, child, elderly person, and the general ailments common to all. The reader is asked to refer directly for this information.

General ailments common to all are:

101 pertaining to the Three Humours:
  Twenty-five Wind disturbances
  Forty-two Bile disorders

Thirty-three Phlegm disturbances

101 principal ailments – there are two divisions or categories:
  (a) Simple
  (b) Complex

101 ailments located in: (a) Body
                        (b) Mind

101 general categories – there are four divisions:
(a) internal ailments from the waist up to the neck
(b) sores
(c) heat disorders
(d) miscellaneous conditions including infections, snake poisoning, infestations and from parasites.

This totals 404 diseases and conditions in all. In addition there is a further sub-classification. There are four categories of disease:

1. Those that result in death even if treated, that is they are incurable, but may be alleviated.
2. Those due to spirits and demons which can be cured through spiritual practice, ritual and exorcism, followed by suitable medication.
3. Illnesses that can be healed but which will result in death if not treated, i.e. they are treatable and generally curable.
4. Self-curing ailments, usually of a minor nature – no treatment is necessary, but treatment may speed up the cure.

The above classification pertains as much to indications for treatment as for diagnosis.

3. The Characteristics of the Illness

The Three Stages of Disease are:

1. Incipient, early stage – symptoms are not clearly manifest.
2. The middle stage when the clinical signs and symptoms are clear.
3. The fully 'ripened' stage when the symptoms are clearly manifest in terms both of their nature and location(s).

The above stages are qualitative; the quantitative aspect is also noted — that is, the relative vigour or feebleness or average force of the disease processes accordingly. These aspects are dependent on and modified by environment, time, biotypology and individual make-up, age, humours, diet and behaviour.

Finally, there are the twenty-five aspects of the soma that can be potentially unhealthy or have pathological consequences as previously mentioned:

(a) Fifteen humours (three × five)
(b) Seven Physical Energies   } = twenty-five
(c) Three Excretory Functions

Hot and Cold diseases relate to the humours as follows:

Wind and Phlegm are cool by nature.
Blood and Bile are hot by nature.
Blood is included as a fourth humour within the context of the further classification of Hot and Cold disease.

Hot diseases are due to an increase in the Bile humour and/or an ebullition of blood, and this results in an imbalance of the Three Humours. Cold diseases are due to an excess of the Phlegm humour. Wind diseases can be either hot or cold depending whether Wind is combined with Bile or Phlegm in the first stage of the disease, although by nature Wind is cold. Ailments due to worms or any organisms in the body, also lymph disorders, are common to both heat and cold. *Fever* is Wind+ combined with Bile+.

Normally body-heat is balanced and as it should be, providing all Three Humours are of equal strength. If one predominates it will be disturbed:

Wind+ causes body-heat to fluctuate, that is feeling hot one moment and cold another.
Bile+ makes it sharp and strong.
Phlegm+ reduces and weakens body-heat.

The genesis of Hot and Cold disorders is explained in the 1st Tantra, Chapter 3:

> Illness comes about by the 3 causes aided by 4 contributing circumstances, resulting in their meeting the 6 types of entrances, and then remaining in the upper, lower and middle portions of the body. Along the 15 Pathways, imbalances of the humours increase in accordance with the 9 conditions falling within the categories of age, environment and time.*
>
> There are 9 conditions any of which result in certain death** and 12 types of reaction imbalances*** of the 3 humours. All these fall into the 2 categories of Heat and Cold.

The above classification of Hot and Cold diseases corresponds to the Yang and Yin of the Tao, which is the basis of Chinese medicine.

The Twelve Types of Reaction Imbalances

1. Bile after curing a Wind disorder.
2. Phlegm after curing a Wind disorder.
3. Bile while still treating a Wind disorder.
4. Phlegm while still treating a Wind disorder.
5. Wind after curing a Bile disorder.
6. Phlegm after curing a Bile disorder.
7. Wind while still treating a Bile disorder.
8. Phlegm while still treating a Bile disorder.
9. Wind after curing a Phlegm disorder.
10. Bile after curing a Phlegm disorder.
11. Wind while still treating a Phlegm disorder.
12. Bile while still treating a Phlegm disorder.

Heat and Digestion[12]

In conclusion, it is stressed by the various Tibetan doctors that the stomach and duodenum is the most important part of the body,

---

* See 'The Classification of Illness' (p. 67).
** See 'The 9 Fatal Conditions' (p. 71).
*** See 'The Twelve Types of Reaction Imbalance' (p. 69).

because all of the life-processes depend on digestion. This function commences principally in these organs. If there is insufficient heat in the stomach the essence of the food will not be absorbed. Dr Pema Dorje and Elizabeth Richards explain the whole process and significance of digestion and maintain the 'digestive heat'.

Dr Tenzin Choedak extends the argument to the health of the foetus in utero – 'a loss of stomach heat could be due to the unsatisfactory diet of the mother'. Dr Trogawa Rinpoche says:

> Body heat causes digestion and this process is dependent on the 2nd Bile humour in the stomach which generates heat and digests food. Almost all parts of the body are pervaded by heat, so if there is the right amount of heat, the nutritive qualities can be extended from the food and absorbed.
>
> Too little heat in the stomach interferes with these functions and:
> (a) reduces the normal capacity to extract nutriment from the food
> (b) interferes with the absorption of the nutriment (essence).
> Too much heat in the stomach increases blood heat and can cause diseases for this reason.

Dr Trogawa Rinpoche says that exceptionally disease can start before digestion in the 'sternum' (most probably in the oesophagus) by blockage and obstruction.

Abnormal Conditions Arising out of the Departure from the Body of its Natural Condition of Health, when the Seven Energies Diminish

1. When the nourishing quality of food (essence) is not absorbed or is only partially absorbed there is: emaciation, swallowing is difficult or impossible, the skin is rough and loud noise causes nausea. This would apply equally to an insufficient intake of food.
2. The blood when deficient (anaemia) causes the arteries and veins to become flaccid, the skin becomes rough and the person takes on a distinctive appearance inasmuch as the body and tissues contract as when very cold.

3. If the flesh loses its strength and tone, there is pain in the joints, and the person has the appearance of being 'skin and bones'.
4. Loss of fat causes pallor and insomnia.
5. If the bones lose their substance (demineralization) the hair, finger-nails and teeth fall out.
6. If the bone-marrow is deficient there is a feeling of 'hollowness' of body and vertigo and cataract can ensue.
7. If potency is diminished or lost many diseases can follow. A cardinal symptom is a burning sensation in the vertebrae.

Abnormal Conditions Arising out of the Departure from the Body of its Natural Condition of Health, when the Three Excretory Functions are Deficient

1. When bowel function is deficient generally Wind is perturbed and rises to the heart.
2. When urination is deficient the person loses the normal colour of the body.
3. When perspiration diminishes the skin cracks and flakes off.

Pathological Consequences

The Nine Fatal Conditions

The nine fatal conditions (incurable illnesses) which lead to biological dissolution (death) are:

1. When the life force is expended – that is, in a natural sense – for example, the natural demise of a relatively healthy person.
2. The situation where as soon as one serious disease is arrested, another takes its place. Irreversible biological dissolution as a result of a long-term pathological evolution. The person is in a terminal state. In a Tibetan medical context this is usually due to the effect of extreme hot and cold conditions.
3. The incapacity of the organism to respond to the usual

medicines or treatment which would normally arrest or reverse the particular illness. Instead, treatment produces the opposite effect, that is aggravation.

4. As a result of trauma and particularly wounding which involves the severance of nerves and blood vessels, or as the Tibetans would say — 'the nerve of life' is cut.

5. When pathological processes have progressed to the point, i.e. having reached a natural limit, whereby they are no longer curable, nor can they be subject to clinical control.

6. In hyperthermia where the temperature is too high and of too long duration (malignant fever).

7. In hypothermia where the temperature is subnormal for too long.

8. Where there is a progressive asthenia (weakening) of the entire metabolism (system).

9. The situation where a demon makes off with the personal energy of the patient, who is usually suffering from what would normally be some controllable or curable condition. Treatment in this instance is totally ineffective.

5

Diagnosis

A discussion follows of some of the problems which, due to the traditional way of teaching clinical application and particularly diagnosis, confront Western students of Tibetan medicine. These are not deemed insurmountable however.

There are distinct difficulties apropos the technicalities and clinical application of Tibetan medicine, both from a diagnostic and therapeutic point of view. The principal difficulty is intrinsic to the traditional mode of training Tibetan doctors, which differs little from the 'oral transmission' basis of Tantric Buddhism. The important and often vital part of the Teachings is passed on directly from Tibetan Master to student, principally in the form of verbal instruction and commentary on the particular text. In traditional Tibetan medicine this means that the medical student is required to memorize the texts by heart.

I have on a number of occasions asked eminent Tibetan physicians the same question – 'Most of the translations made so far of the rGyud bZhi are principally of the relatively short first Tantra and to some degree the second, but why is it that no one seems to want to tackle the long third Tantra, which one is given to understand contains the really essential practical and clinical applications of the theory?' The answer is always the same. Without a prolonged period of what is virtually a clinical apprenticeship during which the limited information conveyed by the written word is interpreted and elaborated on, in the actual clinical situation under the constant supervision and direction of the master physician, mere translation is meaningless. This is why, it would seem, that apart from a few chapters which deal with specific topics, the bulk of the third Tantra has as yet not been translated.

However, thanks to those Tibetan doctors who fortunately for us are spending more and more time in the West, an increasing amount of technical and practical information is being made available. The efforts of English-speaking amchis such as Dr Lobsang Rapgay, with their wide understanding of Western medicine, are particularly helpful to aspiring students in the West. For example in the chapter on Tibetan urinalaysis I have been able to draw on material hitherto unavailable to the non-Tibetan language scholar. I am grateful to Dr Rapgay in making this information available in the first instance in *Myrobalan* no. 3. (see Appendix 1)

Moreover it would seem that distinct possibilities are opening up for clinical training and instruction in the West by qualified Tibetan physicians in a more permanent teaching situation which augurs well for the future at least.

Diagnosis

The principles of continuity, interdependence and relativity are more than evident in Tibetan medical diagnosis. Etiology merges progressively with pathology, which likewise leads without interruption into diagnosis and prognosis, and similarly terminates with treatment in an unending stream. But life and all its processes are like a river, a constant flow of motion without beginning or end. Indeed 'since beginningless time' is mentioned frequently in the Mahayana Sutras.

What has this to do with diagnosis? The previous chapter by no means lists all the etiological factors, pathological consequences and possibilities in the very considerable detail as they are found in the texts themselves. Nevertheless all these need to be actively borne in mind at the point where the practitioner sees the patient and especially at the first consultation. Normally it is then that the diagnosis is made, which is totally 'holistic' for the Tibetan physician. Every factor and aspect is seen as evidence of an imbalance in the total cosmo, psycho-physical sense, and in terms of the philosophy explained more specifically in the Root Tantra and described in the foregoing chapters. Cause and effect operate on every level – horizontally, vertically and in combination. Nothing is unrelated and should it appear to be, it is only apparently by chance.

Method of Clinical Procedures

Classically Tibetan medicine says that inspection, palpation and interrogation, skilfully and competently carried out, will provide all the necessary information about ill health and disease. These procedures are usually carried out in the following order:

1. *Inspection* – consisting of two principal aspects:
   (a) firstly, visual examination of the tongue, and
   (b) secondly of the urine.
   (c) Additionally, with small children, examination of the veins of the outer ears is carried out. Observation of the biotypology comes within this section.
2. *Palpation* – diagnosis by touch is principally concerned with 'taking the pulses', in a similar but somewhat different way from the Chinese and Indian (Ayurvedic) procedures. Within this section generally body tissues are always felt as and when necessary.
3. *Interrogation and listening* – according to the twenty-nine classical questions, plus ascertaining any other possibly relevant information. This listening also involves taking note of the patient's voice in terms of what is said, how it is said, and appreciating any relevant and significant subtleties associated with the vocal function.

N.B. Disturbances and their relevancies of *body*, *speech* and *mind* in the traditional Buddhist context and as they may affect health are therefore fully appreciated by the Tibetan doctor. Classically, there are thirty-eight aspects of diagnosis.[1]

1 Visual Diagnosis

A The Tongue

The three characteristic appearances of the tongue, corresponding to the three humours, making three distinct clinical pictures:

- (a) Wind — red, dry and rough, pimples around the edge, de-hydrated
- (b) Bile — yellow coating, dirty looking, bitter tasting
- (c) Phlegm — coated with phlegm, grey in appearance, soft and 'waterlogged'.

B The Three Humours

- (a) Wind — watery, bluish-white, with bubbles when stirred
- (b) Bile — red, bile coloured (this indicates a Hot Bile disease), thick, strong smelling and steamy
- (c) Phlegm — clear, minimal steam and odour, but frothy.

C The Earlobes

Look into the light from behind at the junction of the ear and the mastoid bone, a yellowish tinge indicates a bile disorder. This is valid in adults as well as children.

D The Eye-lids

In blood disorders they appear red in colour, in hot bile disorders yellow in colour, in cold phlegm disorders pale and white in colour.

2. Pulse Diagnosis (Sphygmology)

This subject is dealt with in the first chapter of the Fourth Medical Tantra. The three characteristic pulses, typical of imbalance of each humour, are found generally as follows:

Wind   – easily compressible and without much tone, can be arhythmic with occasional 'dropped-beats' (extra systoles), generally nervous and 'jumpy'.

Bile   – rapid, wiry, full and feels taut (in Chinese medicine – Yang).

Phlegm – weak, slow and easily compressed – generally 'sluggish' (in Chinese medicine – Yin).

Apart from this brief description, pulse diagnosis is dealt with in depth by Dr Yeshi Donden's translation. Herewith a summary of the thirteen sections:

1. Observances for the patient to follow so the pulse can be determined.
2. The time of the pulse diagnosis reading.
3. The anatomical position for reading the pulse.
4. Pressure exerted by the fingers for taking the pulse.
5. The method by which the pulse is to be interpreted.
6. Three constitutional pulses. The constitutional pulse is present regardless of health or illness but is only read in a healthy person.
7. The reading of the pulse in relationship to the four external seasons and the five internal cosmo-physical energies.
8. Seven divination pulses which are of prognostic importance.
9. The differences in pulse beats in health and disease.
10. General and specific pulses.
11. Death pulses.
12. External force and evil spirit pulse.
13. Lifespan pulse.

As with urinalysis there are similar controls which if not observed can lead to false conclusions. The pulse reading is ideally performed in the morning.

It is traditional to palpate the radial artery on each wrist which is situated at an ideal distance from the organs concerned. Palpating arteries more proximate or distal to the organs tends to lead to distortion of the signals. The palpating fingers of both of the doctor's hands are employed in taking the pulse. There is a traditional way of taking the pulse with both the patient and the practitioner sitting facing one another. Usually the operator's right hand palpates the patient's left radial pulse and vice versa. The pressure exerted on the pulse is variable according to the palpating fingers used (and obviously the organ pulses being palpated). Basically the indexfinger pressure is light and superficial, that of the medius is slightly increased in order to actually feel the flesh, whilst the ring-finger palpates more deeply so that the bone is felt. There are a total of twelve pulses. In male patients the left wrist is 'read' first and with the female vice versa.

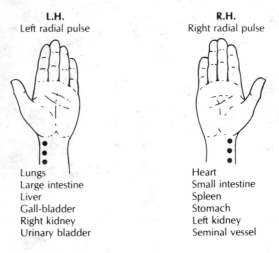

L.H.
Left radial pulse

R.H.
Right radial pulse

Lungs
Large intestine
Liver
Gall-bladder
Right kidney
Urinary bladder

Heart
Small intestine
Spleen
Stomach
Left kidney
Seminal vessel

Figure 2   *The radial pulse*

Apart from the direct diagnostic possibilities in evaluating organ function/dysfunction, other more novel aspects convey interesting and helpful information to the diagnostician. For example:

(a) the three constitutional pulses which particularly relate to life span, family antagonisms and the sex of progeny. The 'bodhisattva pulse' is characteristic.
(b) the important variations on the pulse reading relative to cosmic energies and the seasons.
(c) the seven 'amazing' pulses are intriguing:

Table 6 Comparative Ayurvedic, Chinese, and Tibetan sphygmology[2]

Ayurvedic pulse placements		Chinese pulse placements		
		Left arteria radialis	Yang Superficial	Yin Deep
Arteria radialis	*Meridians*			
Index	Vata	Index	small intestine	heart
Medius	Pitta	Medius	gall bladder	liver
Ring	Kapha	Ring	urinary bladder	kidneys
The pulse is checked on the right wrist of a male while for the female, it is checked on the left wrist.		*Right arteria radialis*		
		Index	large intestine	lungs
		Medius	stomach	spleen
		Ring	'triple warmer'	'heart governor'

Tibetan Sphygmology

Left arteria radialis		Parenchymateous (upper placement)	Hollow Organs (lower placement)	Cosmic energy	Seasonal pulse	Seasonal days
Patient	*Physician*					
female	right index	lungs	large intestine	Metal (Space)	Autumn	72
male	right index	heart	small intestine	Fire	Summer	72
either	right medius	spleen	stomach	Earth	In-between	18
either	right ring	left kidney	reproductive organs	Water	Winter	72
Right arteria radialis						
female	left index	heart	small intestine	Fire	Summer	72
male	left index	lungs	large intestine	Metal	Autumn	72
either	left medius	liver	gall bladder	Wood (Air)	Spring	72
either	left ring	right kidney	urinary bladder	Water	Winter	72

Just the index fingers are switched for the male and the female patients. This is because the energies at the tip of the heart are more concentrated to the right of the female while for the male they are concentrated more to the left.

1. Guest pulse.
2. Family pulse.
3. Enemy pulse.
4. Friend pulse.
5. Evil spirit pulse.
6. Reversing (role) pulse.

The inference, particularly with pulses 1–4, is the existence of a close and empathic rapport between members of the family unit themselves, plus guests. The head of the family (or clan) is the principal point of reference in the pulse-taking procedure.

The evil-spirit pulse (no. 5) demonstrates successful attack on the patient by demonic influences and is very characteristic. The reversing (role) pulse (no. 6) is based on close family ties, and a member of the family can substitute examination of his or her pulse for another relative's pulse, i.e. where the patient cannot be examined directly by the physician because the circumstances prevent it. In addition there are pregnancy pulses, pulses in health and disease, general and specific pulses and the death pulse.

In conclusion, the writer's experience is fully in accordance with Dr Barry Clark's[3] (Tibetan medical) view – the technique of pulse-taking is difficult to master. One really needs constant supervision from a Tibetan doctor and it takes about three years to master it. However there is one consolation. Since Chinese acupuncture has been widely taught and practised in the West, numerous students of the Chinese pulse-taking technique have, with diligence and practice, successfully achieved proficiency. Apropros of the subject of Chinese acupuncture Table 6 (p. 79) shows the comparative Ayurvedic, Chinese and Tibetan pulse placements. As it will be seen, pulse diagnosis is not exclusive to Tibetan and Chinese medicine – it is intrinsic to Indian Ayurvedic[4] medicine too (see Chapter 13).

According to Lobsang Rapgay, relying solely on a pulse reading would be unsatisfactory. Generally the pulse diagnosis relates only to the symptomatic level – a pulse diagnosis therefore reflects only a symptom diagnosis. The ability to relate pulse findings to organic causes and conditions through either pulse diagnosis (or urinalysis) on its own is very difficult.

I am indebted to the Tibetan Medical Institute, Dharamsala, for permission to reproduce the twenty-nine questions relating to disturbances of the Three Humours, and also Table 6 on p. 79.

3. Interrogatory Diagnosis

There are twenty-nine questions relating to disturbances of the Three Humours:

Questions pertaining to Wind disorders:

1. Texture of foods taken — light or rough.
2. Sleep deprivation. — Contributory factors
3. Being exposed to Wind.
4. Going through much suffering.

5. Frequently yawning, trembling, stretching, shivering.
6. Pain in the hip-joints, lumbo-sacral area and all joints, intermittent shooting pains. — Symptoms
7. Involuntary twitching and movement, fidgeting.
8. Reduced feeling and mental instability.
9. Are all symptoms worse when hungry? — Aggravation and
10. Do oily and nutritious foods relieve? — Amelioration

Questions pertaining to Bile disorders:

11. Acrid and hot foods, exposure to hot sun. Losing temper and violent behaviour. — Contributory Factors

12. Bitter taste in mouth.
13. Headaches.
14. Excessive body-heat. — Symptoms
15. Shooting pains in upper part of body.
16. All symptoms worse whilst food is being digested. — Aggravation and
17. Relieved by cool food and environment. — Amelioration

Questions pertaining to Phlegm disorders:

18. Heavy and oily foods. } Contributory
19. Lying on damp ground.   Factors and Aggravation

20. Uncomfortable fullness in stomach.
21. Digestive difficulty generally.
22. Regurgitation.
23. Food has no taste.
24. Distension – meteorism.
25. Belching.   } Symptoms
26. Heaviness of body and mind, lethargy.
27. Body feels chilled, both outside and inside.
28. Discomfort after eating.

Questions pertaining to Phlegm disorders
29. Warm food and environment } Amelioration

Clinical Objectives

(a) Determine the conditions and
    circumstances which led to the
    disease.
(b) Ascertain food habits before the   } Etiology
    present illness.
(c) Ascertain the nature of the present
    diet, that is, since the illness.
(d) Assess and classify symptoms. } Symptomatology

The thirty-eight aspects of diagnosis are sometimes supplemented by:

(i) Astrological diagnosis;
(ii) Dream analysis;
(iii) A type of Iridology;
(iv) Divination.

Tibetan Medical Urinalysis

A very detailed and comprehensive article on the subject particularly addressed to professional health practitioners was published in *Myrobalan* no. 3, November 1985. A reprint of this will be found in Appendix 1. The following summary of procedures represents a useful clinical outline and general framework within which the practitioner can fill in the details, according to the needs of the particular patient being investigated:

General Objective

(a) Assessing the state of health, i.e. what should be normal for that patient, and thus noting any departure from that state; establishing the presence of any degree of organic pathology (if present), and making a prognosis.

(b) The examination of the urine is basic to every patient seen and is usually repeated on each visit and sometimes daily.

(c) The four basic procedures are:
   (i) physical examination;
   (ii) visual examination of deposits;
   (iii) re-examination – looking for change;
   (iv) testing for diagnostic purpose and for selecting the treatment.

(d) Duly noting variables resulting from: dietetic factors and fluid intake, activities, temperature and climate, diuretic medicines, stress, etc.

(e) Instituting controls in order to avoid (d).

(f) Ensuring the proper collection of urine samples in *suitable* containers together with an acceptable stirring stick.

(g) Ensuring the suitable time for collection and examination.

(h) Procedures of analysis generally consist of making a general classification of the urine in terms of the 'Three Urines' typically – rLung, Phlegm and Bile (see above):
   (i) *Principal characteristics on inspection*
       Colour, Odour, Cloudiness and Bubbles.
   (ii) *Examination of deposits*
       Principally sediments and the presence of 'cream'.

(iii) *Examination of urine after change*
Time when change occurs, the way change occurs and post-change qualities.

(iv) Comparative assessment of normal and simple pathological urine, with differential diagnosis.

(v) Similarly for complex pathological urine.

(vi) Differential diagnosis: inflammatory and non-inflammatory disease, specific visceral involvements, determining the acuteness or chronicity of a disease process, assessing the functional or structural emphasis in the clinical problem, indications of allergy.

(vii) Recognizing typical urines, e.g.: of the common cold, meningitis, intestinal colic, enteritis, dyspepsia and weak digestion, flatulence, hepatitis, acute cholecystitis, cholelithiasis, intestinal parasites, pneumonia, bronchitis, asthma, functional or organic heart disease, anaemia, arthritis, tumours.

(viii) Terminating the final examination of the urine in terms of a major differential diagnosis, i.e. summing-up.

(ix) Miscellaneous factors to be borne in mind: the humoural constitutional predisposition and seasonal factors.

(x) Tests for poisoning.

(xi) Tests for determining lines of treatment.

(xii) Dr Rapgay's conclusion: 'No amount of literature on urinalysis can substitute the importance of studying the technique under a competent physician' (Tibetan of course).[5]

It will be seen that the examination of the urine according to the Tibetan medical tradition is a basic routine. In a similar way to the osteopath who carries out both a structural and functional re-examination of the patient on each visit, so it is with the Tibetan doctor who re-examines the patient's urine.

Methodology and Diagnostic Conclusions

Firstly, ascertain whether a disease manifestation is Hot or Cold; the former is usually associated with Bile and the latter with Phlegm; Wind has cool power but can be either Hot or Cold. Disturbances of the Three Humours are not easy to evaluate, systemic as well as localized disturbances often co-exist, and combinations of imbalances can be diverse and complicated. Then follow and apply the three procedures in diagnosing disease:

(i) On the basis of secondary cause factors (nutrition and behavioural patterns).

(ii) On the evaluation of the symptoms presented which indicate the characteristics peculiar to each humour, that is in terms of humoural imbalance, sense organs, urine, tongue, sites of disease, locality, seasons and modalities.

(iii) Diagnosis based on inference drawn from the patient's reaction to food, behavioural stimulus, medicine and therapy.

In conclusion, the entire examination in terms of ascertaining the interruption of balance and disturbed equilibrium as applied to the individual patient, taking into account the biotypology in relation to the total cosmo-terrestrial environment. It will be realized that clinical assessments can be exceedingly complex in terms of all the above mentioned factors and aspects.

Symptomatology

It will be appreciated that in terms of the constitutional and functional background and nature of Tibetan medicine that symptomatology within this context includes most of the 'subjective' symptoms familiar to Western medicine. While these are commonly referred to as being 'psychosomatic' in origin, osteopathic medicine in common with Tibetan medicine is also able to ascribe physical causative factors, i.e. quite apart from any primary involvement of the psyche (see Chapters 14, 15 and 16).

Biotypology in Tibetan Medicine[6]

Predominant Characteristics in:

Wind nature — dark complexion, stooped, feels cold very much, knee-joints 'crackle', is aggressive, argumentative and wants to fight.

Bile nature — florid-yellowish complexion, feels heat very much, is aggressive and intelligent.

Phlegm nature — pale complexion, overweight and carries superficial fat, holds head very upright, is averse to movement, is voluble but never gets angry when arguing, for example.

Morphological and Temperamental Characteristics of the Biotypes

1. The above tendencies as far as these morphological and temperamental characteristics are concerned are inherited and represent a certain type of constitution, which is influenced by the diet and behaviour of the mother during pregnancy. They will be present to a greater or lesser degree.
2. Biotypes are not always pure as such. There can be a predominance of one humour only, or of two humours combined. Sometimes there is even a predominance of the Three Humours, in which case the person is usually very sickly.
3. The Three Humours normally have their own particular relationship and balance. They are linked together so as to allow seven natural 'balances' or combinations, i.e. in health they have their own particular balance.
4. Body colour is not a reliable indicator of humoural balance, rather it should be based on height and build, appetite, character and personality.
5. The predominant humour(s) tend to determine the type of disease or ill health tendencies.
6. Humoural balance is ultimately determined in utero.
7. Variations occur for ethnological and geographical reasons.

6

Mind and mental disorders

Tibetan medicine is primarily functional and physio-pathologic in its approach, based as it is on the humoural concept and the five cosmic energies theory. No distinction is made between physical and mental disorders. The essence is that all life phenomena manifest and express themselves on the one level, through the psychic centres and channels which are equally involved, regardless of the problem. In the case of mental disorders along with 'spirit possession', the Wind humour is particularly involved. The study of mental disorders, therefore, involves at the same time a study of the behaviour of Wind. Everything that has been said pertinent to the psychic channels and the humours in Chapters 2, 3 and 4 equally applies.

It is interesting to note, within this context, a contemporary Western definition of pain – 'Pain is an emotional response to an afferent input'. This is made very clear by Lobsang Rapgay:

> Tibetan theory holds that mind*, consciousness and Wind can all be described along a continuum of corporeality, from the grossest and most physical to the subtlest and most ethereal. Mind, for instance, is described in terms of the gross faculties of physical sensation, the subtle mind that continues into the intermediate state,** serving as the foundation for the next birth. Wind is categorised along the same continuum, physical to subtle to very subtle.[1]

* i.e. specific type of mind (primary or secondary)
** the Bardo

The Nature of the Mind

The study of the mind and its true nature in Buddhism is the subject of two major approaches:

(a) High Yoga Tantra – Mahamudra, Dzogchen, and
(b) the Abhidharma.

The former is concerned with advanced meditational practices and the subtle states of consciousness associated with it. The latter is as the Ven. Chögyam Trungpa Rinpoche says:

> Abhidharma is a survey of the psychology of the human mind. It is part of the basic philosophy of Buddhism, common to all schools – the Theravadins, the Tibetans and so on. . . . The abhidharma is part of what is called the tripitaka, the 'three baskets' or 'three heaps'. These are the three bodies of teaching that constitute the Buddhist scriptures.

Rinpoche gives the subject a contemporary twist:

> Many modern psychologists have found that the discoveries and explanations of the abhidharma coincide with their own recent discoveries and new ideas; as though the abhidharma, which was taught 2,500 years ago, had been redeveloped in the modern idiom.
> The abhidharma deals with the five skandhas. The skandhas represent the constant structure of human psychology as well as its pattern of evolution and the pattern of evolution of the world. The skandhas are also related to blockages of different types – spiritual ones, material ones, emotional ones. An understanding of the five skandhas shows that once we are tuned into the basic core of egohood, then anything – any experience, any inspiration – can be made into a further blockage or can become a way of freeing ourselves. Abhidharma is a very precise way of looking at mind. Any tendency of mind, even the subtlest suggestion of a tendency can be viewed with great precision – even something as slight as the irritation from having a fly perched on one's leg. That irritation, for example, might be classified as a friendly one

which merely tends to frighten the fly away or an aggressive one which moves to kill it.

The abhidharma deals very precisely and impartially with our particular type of mind and it is tremendously helpful for us to see our mind that way. This does not mean being purely scholarly and intellectual. We can relate to little irritations like the one of the fly as just the sort of happening that makes up the human situation. We do not particularly make a big deal about it, but we see it precisely. This eventually becomes very helpful. It is helpful not only for pure meditation but also meditation in action. The whole approach of Buddhism is oriented towards dealing with everyday life situations rather than just meditating in order to attain enlightenment. Throughout the three pitakas there is very little emphasis on enlightenment. The pitakas are handbooks of how to live in terms of the awakened state of mind, but very much on the kitchen-sink level. They are concerned with how to step out of our usual sleepwalking and deal with actual situations. The abhidharma is a very important part of that general instruction.[2]

Mental Illness

Doctors Lobsang Rapgay and particularly Terence Clifford, who is a psychiatrist, have devoted much time to the subject of mental illness and have recorded much in writing. Indeed as Terence Clifford says in the preface of her book, 'This work represents an effort to introduce Tibetan Buddhist medicine in psychiatry in a general way. It began as an inquiry only into Tibetan medical psychiatry but grew into a larger work when all the elements of Tibetan psychiatry took it in expanded directions.'[3]

In view of the expertise reflected in the writings of both Lobsang Rapgay and Terence Clifford, I shall do no more than quickly summarize a few of the important features of this aspect of Tibetan medicine.

Dr Lobsang Rapgay list seven types of madness:

1. With a primary disturbance of Wind;
2. With a primary disturbance of Bile;

3. With a primary disturbance of Phlegm;
4. With a complex disturbance of all three;
5. Primarily characterized by depression (psychotic);
6. Primarily due to toxic causes;
7. Primarily due to harmful spirits.[4]

Causes

Terence Clifford puts it another way and says:

> According to both Abhidharma and the medical tradition there are five causes of insanity:
> 1. Karma
> 2. Grief-worry
> 3. Humoural imbalance
> 4. Poisons
> 5. 'Evil spirits'[5]

Treatment

There are three approaches in psychiatry:

1. Magico-Religious – tantric and yogic practices – exorcisms.
2. Organic – by medicines and other somatic treatments for humoural imbalances and poisons.
3. Psychological – Dharma.[6]

Theodore Burang states: 'The general and basic cause of mental illness is thought to lie in leading a life that runs counter to one's deepest spiritual inclinations and insights and one's inherent disposition'.[7]

In contrast when talking of mental health, Dr Lobsang Rapgay says, 'Mental health is defined as a mind freed from the influence of the afflictive mental factors, and that is the goal of the process of meditation'.[8]

The Ven. Trungpa Rinpoche has evolved a unique method of Dharma psychiatry based on helping recovery within the home environment. This is known as Maitri therapy, and is summarized in a monograph published by Maitri Psychological Services.[9]

7

Ecology and Tibetan medicine

Very much to the forefront these days, ecology is a word that is on everybody's lips. Ecological disasters and iatrogenic disease go hand in hand and are now commonplace manifestations of *homo sapiens'* inability so far to successfully relate and co-operate with nature. People mostly forget their interdependence upon, and place alongside, the amoeba in the pond and cloud in the sky. Ecological disasters concern principally the outer or greater, and to a lesser degree the immediate environment, over which ordinary individuals have little or no control except, in democracies, through their elected political representatives or other public corporate bodies. These may or may not act in their interests and often seemingly poignant issues are ignored altogether. The very existence of private organizations dedicated to ecology emphasizes that individuals are neither very happy nor indeed satisfied with the policies and efforts of the official guardians of public health in this domain, and demonstrates the need for lay vigil and action.

Iatrogenic Disease

Iatrogenic disease is another form of man-made ecological disaster, and in case feminists may object to 'man-made', unfortunately in matters of ecology and its aberrations, it is principally males who make the decisions.

Iatrogenic disease or disease caused by treatment relates specifically to the milieu intérieur (C. Bernard) or the Internal

91

Environment, i.e. both metabolism and 'terrain' (or 'soil', i.e. the constitution of the individual). Fortunately, at this level the individual has full control and choice, for no one, again in a democracy, is obliged or can be forced to take in *per oram* or submit to parenteral injection any substance, therapeutic or otherwise. Where the individual is incapable of making his/her own decision for any reason, such as age or disability, a responsible relative or other person takes the decision for him/her. In the UK not even forced-feeding is normally allowed by law.

Essentially, therefore, people only develop iatrogenic disease by personal decision. Why then are people willing to court disaster for their own bodies? There are three principal reasons it would seem:

1. Fear of disease and fear of death, the latter form being particularly strong in Western cultures.
2. Faith in the doctor or practitioner administering the treatment.
3. Culture and custom in the particular society.
4. Ignorance of complementary treatments available.

Buddhism and the Subject of Death

Fear of disease and death are particularly linked together, and their motivation is very complex and has roots at all levels of human existence. Many volumes have been written on the subject from a biological, psychological, cultural and spiritual point-of-view. The Buddhist approach to these topics has brought solace and peace of mind to many millions of folk past and present in the world, as indeed have other religions and philosophies. The teachings of the *Bardo Thötröl*, the *Tibetan Book of the Dead*, and of Pho'wa, the sixth yoga of Naropa, reveal that at death an individual is able to transfer his or her consciousness to a Buddha-land and, if sufficiently realized, take a future rebirth of one's own choice. These are practical techniques in the art of dying, that can be learned only from a Tantric Master and practised with his permission and guidance.

Therapeutic Faith

It has been said that faith can move mountains. Such is the power of faith, and therapeutic faith is the very first ingredient for healing and recovery from disease. Indeed faith-healers rely totally on faith and nothing from without, sometimes with no mean results to their credit.

Faith in the doctor or practitioner is therefore normal and desirable and to be encouraged. Consequently, it behoves everyone to take an active and positive interest and responsibility for their own health and treatment according to their ability and, hopefully, self-confidence to do so. Where they are unable to do this they must be helped, but normally on the condition that they are agreeable and willing to accept help. Taking a positive interest must not be confused with a negative neurotic and morbid interest. Unfortunately, taking personal responsibility may engender problems but here again help and health education is the key. Nor is angry revolt based on negative emotionalism against the doctor and his drugs the answer either. If you are worried about drug therapy, seek his or her co-operation and discuss your concern, not forgetting that doctors are also worried about iatrogenesis too. Remember the choice is wider in the heterodox or complementary medical field. Be positive and not negative, not only concerning your own health and wellbeing but the general wellbeing and happiness of those around you, too.

Conclusions

Incidentally, it is not only allopathic drugs that can be potentially iatrogenic. Unskilled manipulation by the unqualified manipulator can be as hazardous as the ignorant manipulation of the mind by the untrained psychotherapist. Fortunately, legislation concerned with the safety of medicines has ensured that in most countries the non-allopathic medicines directly available to the public are not able to cause iatrogenic disease, even if prescribed by the untrained 'medicine man'. Whether they will do any good if not skilfully prescribed is of course another matter.

So much for the subject of the ecological disasters involving both macro and micro-environments – commonplace and a great source of worry and concern even for survival in this day and age. But is the subject of ecology something entirely new and pertaining solely to the twentieth century? Apparently not – the subject is, so to speak, almost as old as the hills!

Early Tibetan Buddhist Medical Texts

Predictions

First mentioned in the seventh/eighth centuries and later in the twelfth century, the subject was dealt with extensively in certain Tibetan Buddhist medical texts. Yuthong Yontan the Younger (AD 1112–1203) (see Chapter 1) predicted that in hundreds of years' time the essences of chemicals and diverse poisons would become current causes of disease. According to Dr Tenzin Choedhak, eighteen different 'new infectious diseases' were predicted to eventually appear, including meningitis and cancer, of which fifty-four types are mentioned in the texts. When the environment is charged with chemicals, nature is disturbed and viruses (' 'bu' – worms, in Tibetan) enter the body and cancer starts. All this was predicted in the past and has been particularly stressed in the present by Dr Choedhak. Excesses of chemicals in the environment with much building construction, mining and industrialization plus stress, says he, can cause major Wind disturbances (the humoural basis of neurosis and nervous diseases), ubiquitous in our time.

Naturally Occurring Poisons

Poisons in many forms from the rays of the sun, moon and stars, poisons under the earth coming to the surface with mining which causes poisoning of the minerals themselves, plus poisoning in the air and environment – all these possibilities were known and predicted.

Two examples of the existence of poisons in plants are Rhus toxicodendron and Aconitum napellus. There are nine poisonous plants to avoid, and allergies can occur due to poisonous irritants in plants. Also there are poisons in the coats and spikes of animals, some of which give off a poisonous effluvum. Malaria (mosquitos) and rabies (dogs) were also mentioned in the texts. Dr Choedhak also mentioned poison in decomposing meat and those created by wrong food mixtures – chicken and yoghourt are an example.

Stress

Due to industrialization and urbanization he said, while we are materially advancing we are by paradox creating illness as a result. Cancer, neurosis and nervous diseases and functional heart disease allied very much to stress were hardly known in Tibet before the Chinese occupation, but particularly since the upheavals of the Cultural Revolution they have become very common, affecting even young children.[1]

John Davidson, MA, in the February 1985 issue of the *Journal of Alternative Medicine*, writes 'How electro-magnetic "smog" affects human energy'. The following excerpt is very pertinent to our subject under discussion:

Modern physics and ancient wisdom
Recent research has indicated that these radio and TV wavelengths, once thought harmless, do in fact have an effect on the bio-physical energy or 'virtual' energy. In nature, one cannot get something for nothing. In order for an electron to exist, there must be an energy blueprint to substantiate it or give it existence in our three-dimensional, physical world. This is the 'ghost' electron or 'ghost' energy out of which our gross, physical world is derived.

This energy blueprint has long been recognized by other cultures. It is the Ch'i of acupuncture, the Prana of yogic philosophy, the subtle or etheric energy vibration of which more and more people are becoming aware within themselves.

The link between this subtle energy and gross physical matter is in the movement and spin of the sub-atomic particles. All sub-atomic particles are in constant motion; they spin and move in three dimensions. One can say that the movement of energy in three dimensions is what makes physical matter 'solid' or 'real'. This physical universe is motion, action – cause and effect – Karma as the Indian yogi philosophers call it.

This spin can be clockwise or anti-clockwise. When it is anti-clockwise, the motion is centrifugal, the energy flees the centre; this leads to decay, degeneration and death. When it is clockwise, the motion is centripetal, the energy seeks the centre. This gives rise to coherence, compression, heat, light and life.

In the physical universe, we observe this interplay in constant motion: duality – birth and death, light and darkness, heat and cold, happiness and sorrow, health and disease, positive and negative – the pairs of opposites, also spoken of in the Bhagavad Gita and Hindu scripture. In high energy physics terms, this duality is created by the direction of spin of the sub-atomic particles, which in turn is created by the polarities in the etheric element of subtle matter.

In the physical world, the flow of subtle energy is experienced as atmospheres or vibrations. In living creatures, its polarities and flow manifest as the state of health and well-being. Hence, an acupuncturist need only balance and harmonize the flow of Ch'i, to create changes in the health and well-being of his patient.

Those elements of life, therefore, that effect subtle energy polarities and flow will affect our health and well-being. That includes almost everything – food, water, air, mental attitude, the presence of other people and – most importantly – electro-magnetic radiations, including those at radio and TV broadcast wavelengths, and emissions from ordinary mains wiring.[2]

Practical Advice

So much for these uncanny and accurate predictions which have so horrifyingly come true – what can be done? Dr Choedhak offers the following practical advice, based on the principles of Tibetan medicine:

(a) Be careful with our diet and behaviour (on the lines laid down in Chapter 8).
(b) Consciously avoid contamination, especially by chemicals as far as it is within our ability to do so.

(c) We must endeavour to 'de-stress' ourselves as much as possible, ideally by meditation and spiritual practice generally.

In a more preventative sense we can gain help from:

1. Tantric practices – it is important to take teachings on Vajrasattva and Vajrapani and do the meditations, visualizations and mantras.
2. Taking prophylactic Tibetan medicines.

Prophylactic Tibetan Medicines

Dr Tenzin Choedhak, Chief Medical Officer of the Tibetan Medical Centre in Dharamsala and Personal Physician to His Holiness the Dalai Lama, after a break of seventeen years in a Chinese prison, on the initiative of His Holiness in 1980 put into production a medicine called Tsothel – which is a purified and de-toxified mercury powder with a sulphur base. Tsothel forms the basis for three important Precious Pills. The recipe for making it is found in the Kalacakra Tantra taught by Sakyamuni Buddha and involves a complicated pharmaceutical process – a kind of 'burning-out' of the toxic agents with the help of sixteen precious minerals and other metals, so that the ensuing products are perfectly safe and have no side effects whatsoever.

Tsothel and precious pills

After the successful completion of compounding the 'Ngochu Tsothel' – purified mercury, sulphur and sixteen minerals and metals, the doctors at the Tibetan Medical Institute made the three Precious Pills, using the Tsothel as a base.

The Tso-tru Dhashel Chenmo or the Precious Purified Moon Crystal was the first precious pill compounded. This pill comprises of about 55 different ingredients and it purifies the blood, helps with the circulation of the blood and combats poisons in the body and treats liver ailments. It is excellent for combating infections and inflammations such as ulcers and is a good tonic for the health. This pill clears all senses and restores the memory and it also prevents wrinkles and white hair.

The Rinchen Mangjor Chemo or the Great Precious Accumulation pill was compounded in the Centre earlier, but this is the first time that it is compounded with the Tsothel. This pill has about 65 different ingredients and it is excellent for combating poisons of all nature and treats old and hidden diseases. It is especially beneficial for combating plant, insect, animal and chemical poisons.

The Rinchen Ratna Samphel or the Precious Wish Fulfilling Jewel is also compounded accurately for the first time out of Tibet. This pill has 70 different ingredients, with the addition of the Tsothel, which has 18 different ingredients; it totals to 88 different substances. This pill controls poisons in the body system, hypertension, strokes, paralysis and all nerve disorders. It is good for heart ailments, cancer and it has also been used for the treatment of tuberculosis.

This latter pill is very popular with the Chinese and of what is made in Tibet, 90% of this pill is sent to China for the use of Chinese officials and even for export to Western countries (as stated by doctors coming out of Tibet).

The above pills are prescribed by Tibetan doctors for cancer. It has proved to help a number of cancer patients and it has been extremely beneficial in relieving pain in advanced cancer patients, though a more thorough research on the benefits of these pills for this special disease can be done in the near future.

The above pills may be taken by a healthy person to prevent illnesses, as a tonic and a rejuvenating agent, especially the Purified Moon Crystal and the Ratna Samphel are very popular. Many sacred pills are mixed in this medicine also and many prayers were said when they were made. The first pill is taken twice or thrice a month and the latter pill is taken once every month or two when one is not sick and more often when one is ill.*

Apart from their more specific indications as mentioned above, Tsothel medicine can be used in health and disease and in a

---

* This extract is an edited extract from literature published by the Tibetan Medical Institute, Dharamsala.

preventative as well as a curative sense. Because of their rejuvenating qualities, the pills are particularly indicated in those chronic conditions caused by poisoning, and are recommended for psychological problems arising from internal disturbances due to negative external energies. The medicine is preventative in combating the effects of environmental poisons.[3]

Dr Choedhak recounted how, starting at the time of the 5th Dalai Lama, and during the period since, 2–300 kilos of precious medicinal gold and silver had been stored in sacks in the Potala Palace. The Chinese Communists found this and threw it all out because it looked just like any old black powder. Most of it went down the latrines. When they realized the significance of what they had done Dr Choedhak was released from prison, where he had been breaking stones for seventeen years and incidentally had had his jaw broken by some brute of a guard, to make precious pills for the Chinese officials.

Meanwhile, His Holiness was keen that the Precious Pills should be available outside of Tibet but there was not a Tibetan doctor in Dharamsala who was able to make them. There was also difficulty in getting together the some seventy ingredients necessary for compounding the pills. The Chinese therefore allowed Dr Choedhak to leave Tibet and go to Dharamsala. The Precious Wish Fulfilling Jewel Pill, one of the series that controls poisons in the body, is good for hypertension, strokes, paralysis and all nerve disorders and is also used for cardiac conditions, cancer and TB, and is very popular with the Chinese. Ninety per cent of the production of this pill is exported to China for the use of Chinese officials and is also available for Western countries.

But again as with the preparation of all Tibetan medicines the processes are not solely pharmaceutical. His Holiness gave Men-la – Medicine Buddha Initiations – with Himself personally doing the prayers for the launching of these Jewel Pill Medicines. It took a team of Tibetan physicians and assistants over a month of almost continuous working to complete the preparation of 54 kilos of Tsothel (please refer to explanatory leaflets published by the Tibetan Medical Institute, Dharamsala).

Conclusion

Nothing new under the sun – not really! 'When the Iron Bird flies and the Horse runs on Wheels, the Tibetans will be scattered like ants across the face of the earth, and the Dharma will come to the Land of the Red Man*' – prediction of Padmasambhava (Guru Rinpoche) in the ninth century.

---

* generally conceded to mean the USA

8

Introduction to treatment

The diagnosis is specific and 'pin-point', and is individual to each patient as is the treatment, which is directed at the patient rather than the disease. In applying treatment it must be borne in mind that there are basically three types of patient and the clinical approach differs accordingly (See 'Biotypology', Chapter 5).

Clinical Problems

There are three types of clinical problems:

1. The seriously ill patient where deterioration is either imminent or in actual progress and treatment is urgent and combative. The problem may be acute or chronic.
2. The chronic and less ill patient, either functional or organic, where the treatment is constitutional, long-term and less urgent. Dr Yeshi Donden says that it's often better to wait until the patient is ready for treatment.
3. Emergencies, which demand the application of urgent, symptomatic and appropriately localized procedures.

Methods of Treatment

1. The 'dpyad' method[1] which has a three-fold classification: 'Jam dpyad' or gentle methods:

    (i) Burning of incense (of which there are some twelve different varieties).

    (ii) The use of herbal medicines orally, sometimes combined with animal and mineral substances, medicinal baths and ointments applied to the skin and sometimes to the nasal passages.

    (iii) Fomentations and massage.

2. 'Risub dpyad' – coarse methods: includes venesection, moxibustion, lancing abcesses, etc.

3. 'Drag dpyad' – violent methods, surgery, curettage, cauterization, burning with hot irons, etc.

Four Categories of Disease

The four categories of disease in terms of severity and suitability for treatment or not, as the case may be, are:

(a) easy to heal – with suitable medicines, good nursing and co-operation on the part of the patient.

(b) difficult to heal – long-term, will require all the physician's skill and probably multi-therapy.

(c) incurable – the physician gives placebos and support while the patient is encouraged to live according to his or her usual life-style during this lifetime.

(d) where treatment is withheld – those who are suffering from the 'nine fatal conditions' (see Chapter 4) – treatment may only hasten their demise.

The Principal Therapeutic Methods

There are a number of different therapeutic approaches. Treatment may consist of specific advice only, while at other times it is combined with different methods, of which the administration of medicine is the most common. Apart from the former behavioural therapy these may be summarized as follows:

1. Medicinal: oral, including purgatives, emetics; ointments and oils applied externally; medicinal baths.
2. Hydrotherapy: hot baths, hot springs (five types), enemas of two kinds: solid medicines and ointments (jam-tzis) and water mixed with medicines (nir-ru-hal).
3. Acupuncture and Moxibustion: for the former gold needles are used (ser-khab) and the latter involves burning applied to certain points on the skin by either herb or heated gold, silver or iron instruments.
4. Massage – either with the hands or hot stones.
5. Use of heat to relieve pain – the heat is induced by friction of a small applicator on wood which is then applied to the specific point of pain – also friction by gold (serme or gsermrai transliterated).

Note Dr Lobsang Rapgay stresses that the mundane level of Tibetan medicine is the material form (Nirmanakaya) and that Tibetan doctors who are neither lamas nor monks principally practise this.

6. *Basic Dharmic medicine – (healing by Tantric ritual)*
   (a) Mantras and ceremonial rites (pujas), particularly for th treatment of emotional problems, associated with certai Deities: the Medicine Buddha; Vajrasattva; Avalokiteshvar: Hayagriva; Vajrapani; Garuda; and Tara.
   (b) Burning Incense (Zimpa).
   (c) Exorcism by a lama in the case of possession by evil spirits, demons and nagas.
   (d) Dharma teaching, particularly by a lama.

Basically the province of the lama is concerned with the karma of the patient and dealing therefore with the root-causes, i.e. the Three Poisons which in their turn aberrate from the normal balance and functions of the Three Humours. Tibetan doctors who are lamas and/or monks are competent to practise both. All lamas practise 6(c) as being intrinsic to their general function of being a lama.

Warning

Practitioners of the other medicines who are constrained to use the philosophy of Tibetan medicine as a practice model for their own therapy(ies) must perforce practise principally in terms of the mundane level, especially if they have not taken formal Buddhist vows and especially Tantric initiation. To attempt to do otherwise, in other words assume the role of a lama, could cause irreparable harm both to themselves and their patients.

This does not preclude simple and effective counselling in terms of the Buddha's basic teachings, which are available to every layman for both personal guidance and sharing with others, quite a different matter from Tantric ritual healing.

In conclusion, Terry Clifford constantly stresses that meditation and Dharma are the ultimate medicines which will enable us to become aware of our inner processes in a whole new way, to allow the liberation of all our feelings and thoughts and the development of a state of natural peace and wisdom.

Classification of Methods of Treatment

Methods of Treatment are thus classified:

1. Jampa Che
2. Trsub dpyad
3. Drag dpyad
4. Nutritional
5. Eliminative
6. Medicines:
   (a) with disease alleviating properties − five principal types: decoctions, powders, pills, syrups, medicated butter
   (b) with eliminative properties − five types: purgatives, emetics, nasal medication, suppositories and by enema.
7. Symptomatic
8. Basic Dharmic medicine by Tantric ritual
9. Radical
10. Psychological

Dr Yeshi Donden advises:

Ailments of a minor nature are treated by dieting and strict adherence to a careful programmed daily routine without medicines. If a patient is suffering from a disease in a medium state of condition decoction is prescribed; in a more advanced case, medicines in the form of pills are administered; in diseases of a serious nature, treatment consists of bloodletting, moxa, administration of medicines (and) use of (the) psycho-therapeutic process to produce emesis, and bathing in hot springs or in hot water treated with medicinal compounds.[2] *Note* Surgery was discontinued in the ninth century AD.

Two Levels of Treatment

In conclusion it may be said that there are two levels of treatment:

1. The fundamental, which involves the Buddha's Three Cures:
   (a) Wisdom-insight cures ignorance and confusion;
   (b) Virtue-compassion cures attachment, clinging, greed and lust;
   (c) Contemplation-meditation cures anger, hatred and aggression.
   The lama and spiritual teacher is the physician on this level.
2. The mundane, whether holistic or superficial and sympto-matic. The Tibetan doctor or practitioners of other medicines are the physicians on this level.

9

Behavioural therapy

This is in two parts by:
1. Dietetic advice
2. Changing unhealthy and/or unsuitable behavioural patterns.

Both procedures if observed by healthy persons, or at least those who are not necessarily exhibiting outward signs of ill health, can be adopted as a preventative and health-maintaining regimen.

1. Dietetic Advice

Broadly speaking this means, in a negative sense, avoiding foods etc. that are known to be inimical to the particular humoural imbalance in the individual concerned. Looking at the same thing positively it means selecting those articles of diet which are known to be beneficial. Foods have a specific action which depends on their inherent qualities. The food contra-indications as applied to disturbances of Wind, Bile and Phlegm generally are summarized in Chapter 4 (page 51 onwards).

Foods are classified thus:
1. Grains
2. Oils
3. Meat
4. Green vegetables
5. Liquid diet   (Rechung Rinpoche)[1]

(a) Wind Disorders

In principle the diet should have a heavy, greasy, soft and warm qualitative basis, and should include such foods as: mutton, horse meat, old meat,* brown sugar and molasses, meat soups, beer (Tibetan), wine made from molasses, wine made from bone, rock-salt, garlic, onion, old butter.*

(b) Bile Disorders

Foods should be cooling in quality.

- (i) *For Hot Bile disorders*: Flesh of mountain animals (goats for example), fresh cow (and goat) butter, curds and whey made from cow and goat's milk, snow water, cool mountain water, cooled boiled water.
- (ii) *For Cold Bile disorders*: Fresh mutton, yak meat, and herbivorous animals generally, fish, buttermilk from cow or goat's milk, fresh butter from the dzo (the calf of a yak and cow that have been cross-bred).

     Generally: Fresh vegetables, light, cool and well cooked. Porridge made from barley that is about to ripen, boiled dandelion leaves.

(c) Phlegm Disorders

- (i) Yellow Phlegm: Mutton, ginger (tea), fish, grains grown on dry land and particularly flour made from old grain, honey.
- (ii) Brown Phlegm: Fish, pork, young goat's meat, whey and curd made from dzo milk, boiled cold water.

     Generally: concentrated 'chang' (Tibetan beer).

As a rule one should avoid stale, sour by age and mouldy foods. Moreover the quantity of food taken per day should be neither too much nor too little. Rechung Rinpoche suggests a good yardstick is that the quantity of food taken in the morning should be such so

* not stale

that one is able to digest it by the afternoon, and the quantity of food taken in the evening is such that one can digest it by dawn.

Moreover, it is obvious that not all of the foods mentioned are either available, or habitually consumed, outside of the Himalayan region, so the advice traditionally given must be adapted to Western conditions accordingly.

Rechung Rinpoche tabulates very useful information concerning food and drink generally in Chapter XVI of his book *Tibetan Medicine*. Chapters XVII, XVIII, XXIII and XXIX are also highly relevant. Chapter XXVII presents an interesting polemic between Nepalese doctor Sri-Simha and gYu-Thog Yontan mGonpo on the relative merits in relation to health of 'Salt, Beer, Sunlight and Women'.[2] The following diversion from the classical discussion is relevant.

Raw Food Diet

When Dr Tenzin Choedhak was in the UK he was interviewed by Cheryl Isaacson of *Here's Health* who, in her article of October 1983, expressed considerable astonishment at his views on raw foods, and the unsuitability of such a regimen in many cases. As she wrote – 'The doctor's views on raw food were surprising, now that the health kick of a salad a day is finally catching on'.

The rationale of Dr Choedhak's argument in this respect is of course based on the fundamental tenet of Tibetan medicine, that all humoural imbalances start in the stomach, i.e. if 'digestive heat' is not maintained (see Chapter 3). To quote further – for general health 'a little of everything in moderation' is what the Tibetan doctor orders. Chinese medicine would also appear to subscribe similarly to the view that hot, cooked food is superior, according to Lizzie Bingley (a British acupuncturist who recently completed a postgraduate course in China).

From a Western food-reform point of view, raw food diet generally has a place but biotypology is a deciding factor. Thin, highly-strung ectomorphs who are biotypologically predisposed to irritable gut problems (analogous to Wind-types in Tibetan medicine) do not handle raw-food diet at all well. The rounder, petite and softer-tissued endomorphs tend to do somewhat better, but only the athletic, heavy-physique mesomorphs really handle raw food well. These remarks do not apply to raw-food fanatics, who in their extremism are not likely to take a 'middle-way' attitude, regardless of the flatus and intestinal discomfort that they may well suffer along with those in their close proximity.

Quite apart from such clinical and aesthetic considerations there are other reasons, both botanical and ecological, why cooked food and particularly that of vegetable origin (including grains and pulses) is not only preferable, but in some instances absolutely essential.

Botanical Reasons for Cooking Food

Principally a matter of neutralizing the toxic constituents of certain plant foods. As Irvine E. Linder says in the Introduction to *Toxic Constituents of Plant Foodstuffs* (1969) – 'Fortunately, cooking and other common means of preparation have proved to be effective in destroying many of the toxic constituents in plant foods.'

These are listed and dealt with under the different headings of protease inhibitors, haemagglutinins, goitrogens, cyanogens, saponins, lathyrogens, etc. It is interesting to note that heat inactivates protease inhibitors. With soybeans for example there is a trypsin inhibitor which is destroyed by heat, thus enhancing the nutritive value. Trypsin inhibitors are also found in the white potato, kidney beans and chick peas. Heat treatment and soaking in most cases generally renders the other listed toxic constituents inactive, i.e. the kidney bean agglutinin is neutralized by heat, ten minutes cooking usually being sufficient. Favism is also discussed at some length.

Large sections of the world's population depend principally on legumes, grains and seeds for their protein requirements, and more and more Western people are eschewing flesh-eating, either for ethical or economic reasons, or both. Thus, it is vital that the processing and preparation of these articles of diet be fully understood, otherwise health may suffer either by deficiency or toxicity.

Ecological Reasons for Cooking Food

These are mainly two in number and are of course related to source, growing methods, type of fertilization (i.e. whether artificial or organic), country in which they are grown or consumed, etc. (environmental factors)

(a) Pesticide content (DDT etc.), i.e. through toxic, chemical sprays, in some countries such as India has reached dangerously high proportions, as indicated by the following extract from *Express Magazine*, Madras, 25 March 1984 – 'KILLING PESTS, POISONING THE FOOD':

> Tests conducted on food samples collected at random from markets in large cities in India have revealed a high percentage of pesticide residues – in some cases in excess of the prescribed tolerance limits. The misuse of highly potent, broad-spectrum pesticides has resulted in high levels of pesticide residues in the food chain whose cumulative effects can do incalculable harm.

What can be done?

> At the consumer level all food stuffs must be thoroughly cleaned by scrubbing and washing before cooking. The peeling of vegetables and fruits has been found to be effective in reducing the levels of pesticides etc. . . . It has also been found that when chappatis are made from maize and wheat-flour, 73 per cent and 80 per cent of malathion residues are lost. Levels of other pesticides such as D.D.T. and B.H.C. (Benzene Hexa Chloride) have also been found to be lowered during cooking.

According to the article, this applies equally to green leafy vegetables. It continues:

> Many health-conscious consumers have become vegetarians on the assumption that they can avoid much of the pesticide residues by eliminating meat, eggs and fish from their diets. Unfortunately, not only wheat, rice and pulses, but vegetables as well, have shown a substantial increase in their pesticide content due to the indiscriminate use of these poisons by farmers on their crops (i.e. in India).

(b) There is a high incidence of amoeba and hepatitis virus-infections, for example, principally endemic in Asia and Africa and particularly in the tropics at one time, more recently common-place in the eastern Mediterranean, and now even the UK is not exempt. How much excessive raw-food consumption in the West may or may not be a contributory factor in the temperate zone, is a moot point. It is certainly old hat that in the Indian Sub-Continent and the Eastern Mediterranean countries consuming raw vegetables and unpeeled fruit, plus drinking the local water (unless boiled and sterilized) is folly, and a certain recipe for amoebic dysentery and hepatitis. These two fairly easily prevent-able diseases are endemic amongst Westerners on spiritual and other pilgrimages in this part of the world, presumably due to fanaticism about 'pure raw-food pulse and grain diet'. An interesting point is that, at one time in Kathmandu, one could always feel absolutely safe eating in Japanese restaurants, even with raw salad, for the simple reason that the vegetables concerned, the cooking-vessels, plates, knives and forks were washed and rinsed in twice distilled, sterilized water. Other restaurants in the city, it would seem, have now adopted similar preventative measures.

The writer of the aricle in the *Express Magazine*, Thankamma Jacob, concludes – 'Of course the best way to get uncontaminated foods is to produce them yourself in your home garden or farm'. It is interesting in this respect that – 'while making the best use of natural controlling factors, such as biological predators, resistant crops and improved cultural methods must be devised'. It is amazing how some of these methods were visualized and stressed in ancient Indian treatises like the Vrkshayurveda of Sagangadhara in the twelfth century. (Chapter 7 on Ecology also stresses the ancient Tibetan viewpoint in such matters.)

In conclusion, it must be said that cooking food is a time-honoured procedure dating back to the discovery of fire. Probably no other activity that involves the basic to the most refined aesthetic sensory gratification (apart from sex), has pre-occupied the human species more than food and drink. An untold number of cookery books bears witness to this and likewise down through the ages viniculture, and the ubiquitous distillation of alcohol from virtually every edible botanic species, in all cultures. All evidence shows that from every point of view – botanical, ecological, physiological, biotypological, gustatory, aesthetically and even medically, in its broadest sense – cooking is on balance not only beneficial, but essential to human health. (Not over- or under-cooking of course.) Balance is the operative word, i.e. between cooked and raw food in the diet. The middle way is obviously the best and right way and the proportion for the individual totally depends on the factors mentioned above and, more particularly, upon temperament and biotypology.

Conclusions

Cooking and eating the foods hot provides:

  (a) the 'digestive heat'
  (b) detoxifies endogenous toxins
  (c) 'neutralizes' pesticides, etc.
  (d) destroys harmful organisms
  (e) softens and renders the food more digestible and in some
       cases actually increases its nutritional value.

With reference to the recommended types of food and drink to be consumed, the instructions given to patients who are taking the Precious Purified Moon Crystal Pills are:

On the day this pill is taken, take no other medicine, and refrain from eating sour food and drinking sour beverages and alcohol. Refrain from taking uncooked grain items, raw fruits and vegetables, garlic and onion, and refrain from intercourse and all strenuous exercises on that day.[3]

2. Changing Unhealthy and/or Unsuitable Behavioural Patterns

As with 'dietetic advice' there are two aspects, the negative and the positive. With the former, again it is a question of avoiding behaviour which is known to be inimical to the particular humoural imbalance in the individual concerned.

Taking a positive view means introducing new life-styles and habits which are known to be beneficial, in terms of the three aspects of behaviour. Chapters 13, 14 and 15 of the Root Tantra deal with these specifically and in considerable detail:

(a) Chapter 13 – continual daily behaviour;
(b) Chapter 14 – seasonal behaviour;
(c) Chapter 15 – occasional behaviour.

(a) Continual Daily Behaviour

This applies to observing healthy activities in relation to body, speech and mind.

(b) Seasonal Behaviour

This means being aware of the different balance of energies during the different seasons, of which there are six (see Chapter 4, page 60), and how they affect the balance of the Three Humours.

(c) Occasional Behaviour

This is concerned with nutrition generally, in terms of hunger and thirst, as well as understanding and giving proper respect to the natural functions of eating, fasting, drinking, vomiting, yawning, sneezing, breathing, sleeping, urination, defaecation, expelling gas and phlegm and spitting. Above all, the eliminatory functions must never be suppressed.

10

Treatment

1. Medication Therapy

(a) Some General Considerations

Beijing Review, the weekly news magazine of the Chinese government, dated 28 December 1981, stated that Tibetan medicine was being studied and developed in Tibet: 'More than 70 per cent of the counties in Tibet have pharmaceutical factories which have now produced 300 kinds of Tibetan medicines' – obviously in accordance with standard Western scientific methods of preparing drugs.

Contrast this report with excerpts and quotations from the Tibetan Medical Institute News-letter of December 1982, issued in Dharamsala:

> H.H. The Dalai Lama presents the Eight Medicine Buddhas. On 22nd July 1982, on an auspicious date and hour; 2nd day of the 6th month, water dog year – Tibetan King's Year 2109, at 1 P.M. His Holiness the Fourteenth Dalai Lama presented the Tibetan Medical Institute with the statues of the EIGHT MEDICINE BUDDHAS.
>
> The Director of the Institute, Mr Lobsang Samden-Taklha, His Holiness's Senior and Junior Physicians, Dr T. Chocdhak and Dr J. Tashi and five doctors and staff of the Institute went to His Holiness's residence to receive the Deities, which were later brought down to the chapel at the TMI Headquarters.
>
> At the Institute the rest of the staff and students welcomed the Deities with scarves and incense and received the blessings

114

of the Buddhas after they were brought in the chapel. Tibetan tea and the auspicious bowl of rice were offered to every member of the Institute after their visit to the chapel.

Eight GYUTHOE monks performed a purification rite in the new chapel and recited the special prayers of the Medicine Buddhas while the NECHUNG monks were invited to make invocations to the Protecting Deities of Medicine and the Protecting Deities of our Leader and Country.

It is further reported:

Preparation of Chungshi Dawoe and Chakchi Dawoe. Second October 1982 coincided with the 15th of the 8th month of the Tibetan calendar. This is the day the atmosphere is at its clearest and purest form in our calendar and when the rays of the moon are strongest. It was a beautiful, clear night and it was an unforgettable experience to be on the roof and view the huge, round, glowing moon arise majestically over the giant dark mountains of Dharamsala.

On the roof of the Tibetan Medical Institute, thirty-five young men and women with their Teacher/Supervisor, Dr J. Tashi, the Assistant In-charge of the pharmacy, Dr Namgyal Tsering and the Director of the Institute, Mr Samden-Taklha gathered to make some special ingredients for medicines of cool nature. The work began with the prayers to the Medicine Buddhas and prayers continued throughout the working period.

Boiled and purified limestone powder is thoroughly grinded and made into a fine paste with milk under the cool rays of the moon. This is then kneaded and made into pancakes and left to be dried in the shade. This Chungshi Dawoe is used mainly for medicines for phlegm disorders of hot nature and for stomach ulcers.

Iron powder and Aru powder (Terminalia chebula Retz.) are mixed with hot water to form a paste. This paste is left for a couple of days until it is brought out in the full moon to be grinded to a very fine paste and kneaded into pancakes. This ingredient is mainly used for stomach ailments, poisoned liver and eye diseases.

Moon light is a cool energy which is required to activate on these cool ingredients and will be used for medicines of cool nature.

Please refer also to the preparation of the Precious Jewel Pills described in Chapter 7.

Dr Yeshi Donden is explicit concerning Dharma and Tantric ritual as being intrinsic and fundamental to the preparation of Tibetan medicinal compounds. He mentions three procedures:

1. Simple compounding (i.e. the actual pharmaceutical preparation – and yes machinery, some very modern, is now used for pulverizing and pill-making in the pharmacy of the Medical College of the Institute – T.G.D.).
2. Intoning mantras to empower the medicines during the process of the compounding. The medicines are thus consecrated and become 'animate from the inanimate'.
3. Tantric ritual preparation which, as he says, requires single-pointed meditation and visualization, whereby the hierophant preparing the medicines becomes the deity and blesses the medicines, and should generate divine pride in being the deity. This is to enhance the curative powers of the medicinal ingredients by psychic means. The principal deities involved in these rituals are: Garuda, Vajrapani and Hayagriva.

There are three stages to this method:

1. Giving the medicines the empowerment directly.
2. Visualizing the medicines as the deity.
3. Visualizing one's self and the medicines as the deity, i.e. one enters the Mandala and identifies with the deity in order to realize the highest state of one's mind. In this instance the practitioner visualizes the Mandala of the Five Jinas (Dhyani Buddhas or Tathagatas) with Men-la the Medicine Buddha, who occupies the first position, i.e. centrally (this is normally taken by either Vairocana or Vajrasattva, according to the lineage or Tantric text in question).

The three stages of preparation correspond with the Nirmanakaya, Sambhokakaya and Dharmakaya respectively and require the practitioner, as with all Tantric practices, to be first empowered and authorized by a lama, who will perform the necessary dbang (wang) – empowerment, and (lung) – oral transmission accordingly. Alternatively of course the ritual can be carried out by a Buddhist monk.

Following on from this it is necessary for the initiate to read and study and seek Teaching on the medical commentaries, and also ideally, says Dr Donden, then go into retreat and meditate.[1]

The ritual preparation aspect has been stressed at some length because of its vital importance. It is the very pith and kernel of the Tantric Buddhist basis of Tibetan Medicine. Moreover it is a far cry from the impersonal, mechanistic conditions under which the 'Tibetan medicines', mentioned above in the Beijing Report, are manufactured under communist Chinese supervision in the best sterile, dialectical materialist tradition.

The first two stages of preparation, quite apart from the Tantric ritual aspects mentioned above, must perforce exclude non-Buddhists, although prayer as understood and practised in other religions could be equally substituted for mantras. For example, for Christians the empowerment of the medicines would come from God. Problems are envisaged though for agnostics, scientific rationalists and non-believers generally.

Recently, in Dharamsala, I was told that many Tibetans in exile prefer medicinal preparations made in Tibet itself, rather than those readily available from the Tibetan Medical Institute in Dharamsala. The reason given was that the medicines coming from Tibet 'work better'. Subsequent reflection on this statement, which was momentarily quite challenging, led to the following conclusions.

A priori – the question must be asked – Is this preference based on any objective evidence clinical or otherwise, or is it simply subjective? If the latter is the case, there are many variables which could account for it. For example:

1. What particular complaints were the more 'successful' medicines being prescribed for? Bearing in mind the great difficulty that practitioners of any school of medicine have, in

determining the degree of psychosomatic element in the majority of complaints that patients present with.

2. Are the medicines in question being personally prescribed after actual consultation with a Tibetan doctor, or on the contrary by proxy, or again are the preparations more or less what we would call in the West 'proprietary', or manufactured to a standard formulae?

With all due respect, are the Tibetan lay-people all that different, if at all, from ordinary folk all over the world, who are primarily concerned with getting rid of their symptoms as speedily as possible? As all practitioners of holistic medicine know, quick results are often no more than a shift of symptoms on a very superficial level, often with no real change in the causal background and the usually present chronic adaptation and compensation which is virtually built-in to the patient's whole make-up. Moreover patients are helped only on the level that they as individuals wish to be helped. Similarly the doctor can only help (or heal as Thinley Norbu says)[2] according to the level of relative truth or situation of causation that he or she is sensitive to and conscious of, in terms of personal spiritual evolution and understanding.

Assuming that the imported medicines in question are being individually prescribed by a Tibetan doctor outside Tibet proper, then it may be that the claim that the imported medicines are more efficacious is therefore substantially true. If not, i.e. if the medicines are being purchased as standard pharmaceutical products, then it may not be true, indeed it may be only a whim!

All these questions would need to be answered before objective conclusions could be drawn. It was suggested that I should be objective and include this additional information in Chapter 6. I have done so and hopefully fulfilled a writer's duty, i.e. to be objective.

This claim would appear on the surface to negate the need for the ritual preparation of medicines – but does it? Not at all – Chapter 2 (pp. 115, 116 and 117) explains why – the ritual preparation is concerned with the pure essence of the medicines, while the pharmaceutical processes deal only with the gross element aspects which influence equally the gross somatic Five-

Element matrix of the physical body. On the contrary, the pure essence of the preparations treat on the pure essence (mind) level of the patient. Within this context Thinley Norbu says exactly the same thing as Dr Yeshi Donden in his teaching, as quoted earlier in this Chapter.

(b)   The Tibetan Materia Medica

The general structure of the Tibetan Materia Medica and the agents traditionally employed consists of:

   (i) Medicinal plants
  (ii) Metals and minerals
 (iii) Parts and products of animals
 (iv) Ordinary or semi-precious stones
  (v) Various forms of salt
 (vi) A few varieties of mushrooms.

(c)   Medicinal Plants

Medicinal plants are evaluated by their taste and, to a degree, their smell — this is relative to their composition in terms of the Five Elements: Earth; Water; Fire; Air; and Space. This evaluation is with reference to the plants' potential therapeutical effect in remedying this or that humoural imbalance.

   (i) mNgar (sweet)   is constituted by Water + Earth
  (ii) Kha-ba (bitter)   is constituted by Water + Air
 (iii) sKyur (sour)   is constituted by Earth + Fire
 (iv) bsKa-ba (astringent) is constituted by Earth + Air
  (v) Tsa-ba (acrid)   is constituted by Fire + Air
 (vi) lan-tshwa (salty)   is constituted by Fire + Water[3]

The Five Elements relate to the growth of medicinal plants and indeed all vegetation as follows: the plants grow in the Earth, they are moistened by Water, warmed by Fire (the heat of the sun), touched by the Wind (air causes movement and exchange of gases, another stimulus to growth), and the sky provides Space for growth. Rechung Rinpoche classifies medicines as being by quality: heavy, smooth, cool, oily, light, rough, warm and sharp. These different qualities either increase or decrease the Three Humours accordingly.[4]

Literature on Tibetan medicines, their qualities both generally and specifically, is quite considerable and suitably detailed. The titles of translated published works and articles, of interest more to health professionals, will be found in the Chapter Notes. Both Terry Clifford's and Dr Bhagwan Dash's books contain parts of the extensive Materia Medica. A very concise and practical Tibetan Materia Medica compiled and translated by Dr Pema Dorjee is now available in English under the title of *150 Tibetan Medicines*, from the Tibetan Pharmaceutical Centre, Ashoka Niwas, McLeod Ganj, Dharamsala 176219, (HP) India.

One contribution that should be particularly mentioned is by Kelsang Rapten B Sc (Biochemistry) of the University of California; it is entitled *Tibetan Medicinal Plants and Their Relationship to Modern Chemical Activity*.[5]

In Chapter 1 of the Root Tantra there are descriptions of the 'City of Healing', said to be near Bodh Gaya, although there are different interpretations as to the actual site. This is called Tanaduk – 'Beautiful to Behold' – a miraculous creation of Buddha Shakyamuni. There, were to be found the five kinds of precious materials: gold, silver, white and red pearls and lapis-lazuli, which radiate the healing light of the five colours – white, yellow, red, blue and green. The text goes on to describe the four mountains proximate to the city:

> to the South – Big-chey, Thunderbolt Mountain
> to the North – Kangchen, Snowclad Mountain
> to the East – Bo-ngay-den, Fragrant Mountain
> to the West – Malaya, Cool Mountain.

Different medicinal plants are found on each mountain, each with their specific qualities and therapeutic indications, relevant to the treatment and cure of the 404 ailments, in terms of Hot and Cold diseases, and other imbalances of the Three Humours.[6]

Contemporary Obstacles to the Use of Tibetan Medicine in the West

Today in Europe 2500 years after the paranirvana of Shakyamuni Buddha, the Medicines Act in the UK and identical EEC legislation have rendered it almost impossible to employ anything but an extremely abridged form of the traditional Tibetan Materia Medica. How banal it all seems!

Import licences and/or manufacturer's licences are required for all compounded products, although herbalists are exempt, providing their mixtures of herbs are prescribed and made up individually for each particular patient. Biological standardization is compulsory and the legislation is very strict concerning the therapeutic use of toxic substances. Not all substances used in Tibetan medicine would necessarily qualify for the classification of 'non-toxic' under the legislation, and therefore be exempt from restricted sale.

This is not to say that a solution to this problem will not ultimately be found. Allied to this is the question — who is going to use and prescribe such medicines? There is at the moment virtually no one, with the exception of several Tibetan doctors living in the West, who are as yet qualified to do so.

On the other hand, whether or not some importation of certain standard formulae medicines for lay consumption may come about, is dependent upon future decisions and arrangement with the Tibetan Medical Institute in Dharamsala. Meantime there are no available compounded and empowered medicines as yet available. The most likely solution, according to Dr Rapgay, lies in the fact that in India, Tibetan medicines are classified by the appropriate authorities as being 'Ayurvedic'. Since a classification already exists for the latter then the same import/export regulations should apply equally to Tibetan medicines. Importation under licence into Western countries may therefore present less difficulties than it was originally thought.

In Chapter 12 the possibility of adapting the practice of physiomedicalism with a Tibetan medicine orientation and utilizing the existing *Botanic Pharmacopoeia* (UK)[7] has been discussed. Some of the basic plant medicines used in Tibetan medicine are also included in this repertory, indeed some are common culinary herbs such as cloves, nutmeg, saffron, ginger, cardamom, black pepper, etc. The particular qualities of the latter, and its traditional usage by monks in Ayurvedic terms, are mentioned in Chapter 13.

2. Accessory Therapy

Methods

These methods may be grouped together according to their nature and clinical use. They have already been discussed in Chapter 8 ('Introduction to Treatment') but are mentioned again and tabulated here, solely for the sake of completeness.

(a)	Acupuncture and moxibustion.	
(b)	Hydrotherapy:	Frictioning the body with cold water, hot-spring bathing — there are five categories of hot springs.
(c)	Humoural therapy (European term):	Venesection, cupping (ventouses Fr.), cauterization with hot irons.
(d)	Forced elimination methods:	Emetic treatment, enemas, inducing nasal discharges (Sna rdzong Tib.).
(e)	Pyretic treatment:	heat treatment using hot stones and sand-packs.
(f)	Massage:	applied by the practitioner to the patient, particularly for old, feeble people — indicated for bad-kan (Phlegm) disorders, mental stress problems. Kum Nye, relaxation procedures to be carried out by the patient or person, is the subject of two volumes, by Tarthang Tulku and is relevant.

It is interesting to note that, apart from Sna rdzong which would appear to be an exclusively Tibetan procedure, naturopaths (and Heilpraktikers in W. Germany) make considerable use of all these accessory therapies. The apparatus used in hydrotherapy and pyretic treatment in the West, particularly in Europe, is of course highly sophisticated nowadays, but that does not necessarily say that the results are superior to those obtained by Tibetan doctors, using very simple and traditional means.

Conclusions

In conclusion, pertinent to the question of whether scientific medicine be superior to empirical traditional approaches, the editorial of *The Times*, 10 August 1984 is quite pointed in its remarks. It talks about 'a growing loss of faith by the public in a purely scientific approach to medicine', indeed it continues with a stronger statement:

> This groping for some extra dimension to health care, however, goes beyond a state of dissatisfaction with hospital waiting lists and crowded clinics. It suggests that many more people are now coming to reject the purely scientific approach to medicine. . . . They (the medical establishment) continue to disregard the personal factor in medicine and prefer to believe that all physical states can be examined and explained objectively.
>
> The personal factor, encompassing a direct and continuing dialogue between doctor and patient, is at the heart of most systems of alternative treatment. . . . Can the medical world, from its laboratories, also recognise that there is an extra dimension to the art of healing which deserves to be more fully integrated into current systems based predominantly on objective observation? It may be a hard and long process, giving birth to much argument, and many rivalries. However, even the Hippocratic Oath recognised that, in certain callings, spiritual quality is as basic as skill.

Verily the wheel of medical paradox in this age – the age of scientific medicine – has turned almost full cycle within a very short period of time. The turning of the Third Wheel of the

Dharma, that of Buddhist Tantra (including medicine), has not ceased in 2500 years.

Does Tibetan Medicine work? This perennial question surrounds any system of medicine, when most of the available literature is principally dealing with theory rather than practice. However, like both the Chinese and Indian systems, Tibetan medicine has stood the test of time. Not much more in terms of objective statement can be said. There is always the personal experience of individuals of course, which is perforce convincing.

Recently, I was in Dharamsala. Feeling distinctly queasy, I consulted Dr Yeshi Donden. Clinical findings showed a Bile/Wind urine and the whites of my eyes were a slight yellow tinge. Three days of dietary restriction plus the appropriate oral medicines quickly restored normality. Of course, one personal experience does not prove anything but I can only say that the relief was both very welcome and highly impressive.

PART TWO

Relating Tibetan Medicine to Western Holistic Systems of Medicine

11

Introduction to relating Tibetan and Western Holistic Medicine

Holism versus Reductionalism

Apart from allopathic medicine, which is mechanistic and reductive in its approach to health and disease and is primarily based on the doctrine of single causation and above all on the germ theory, other heterodox medicines are all basically holistic and accept that causes may be multiple.

What is meant by 'holistic'? Fritjof Capra[1] puts it succinctly – 'The term "holistic", from the Greek – "holos", refers to an understanding of reality, in terms of integrated wholes whose properties cannot be reduced to those of smaller units'.

Reductionism on the other hand is, as he says, based

> on the mathematical theory of Isaac Newton, the philosophy of Rene Descartes and the methodology advocated by Francis Bacon. . . . Matter was thought to be the basis of all existence, and the material world was seen as a multitude of separate objects assembled into a huge machine. Like human-made machines, the cosmic machine was thought to consist of elementary parts. Consequently it was believed that complex phenomena could always be understood by reducing them to their basic building blocks and by looking for the mechanisms through which these interacted. This attitude, known as reductionism, has become so deeply ingrained in our culture that it has often been identified with the scientific method. The other sciences accepted the mechanistic and reductionistic views of classical physics as the correct description of reality and modeled their own theories accordingly. Whenever

psychologists, sociologists, or economists wanted to be scientific, they naturally turned toward the basic concepts of Newtonian physics.

In the twentieth century, however, physics has gone through several conceptual revolutions that clearly reveal the limitations of the mechanistic world view and lead to an organic, ecological view of the world which shows great similarities to the views of mystics of all ages and traditions. The universe is no longer seen as a machine, made up of a multitude of separate objects, but appears as a harmonious indivisible whole; a network of dynamic relationships that include the human observer and his or her consciousness in an essential way.[2]

There is thus already a common meeting ground with Tibetan medicine. I well remember a discussion I had with Dr Yeshi Donden in his Clinic in Dharamsala. We chatted very generally about diverse clinical matters and I was struck by the similarity of our own particular viewpoints in so many instances. At that point in time I knew almost nothing about Tibetan medicine, yet here I was finding many points of common agreement in a discussion that was so familiar it could have been taking place in my school. In the intervening years I have learnt more and more about the subject, only to be frequently amazed by the similarities I have come across. It has been said that no knowledge is really new, one only re-discovers the old and perennial and gives it new form and concept. So, not only is there a common meeting ground for Eastern and Western medicine, which in itself is a starting-point – i.e. a basic common view – but this is of course once again expressed in very different terms.

First of all, there are the immediate and short-term causes of disease, which require what one might call the Inner-Form Medicines. That is, those where the diagnostic and therapeutic stimuli are directed particularly to that vibrational and bio energetic level. This would seem significant, particularly when considering homoeopathy, and also herbal medicine, with regard to the astrological conceptual model of the early herbalists such as Culpeper and Gerard.

Patterns of imbalance are also very important, as are normal patterns of balance, reflecting constructive adaptation and compensation. Dr Aubrey Westlake wrote an important book on the subject some twenty years ago – *The Pattern of Health* (London, Vincent Stuart Ltd, 1961).

Energy Fields

Again in a Western context the work of Burr and Northrup[3] on the *Electro-Magnetic Pattern-Body and the 'L' Fields – the energy fields of living organisms* is extremely relevant. They showed that the 'L' Fields were continuous, mostly cyclic variations that coincide with the circadian rhythms, sunspot cycles, and lunar environmental, behavioural, psychosomatic factors, and secondly, the common acceptance that disease results from the disruption of the homeostatic mechanisms with ensuing imbalance. Moreover that health is wholeness of body, speech and mind.

The notions of embryolgy, anatomy and pathology in Tibetan medicine, as we have seen, are not necessarily identical and for the good reasons Elisabeth Finckh has already stated (see Chapter 3).

Diagnosis, as we already understand, is functionally based and is directed at assessing physiopathology rather than pathology as such. In this respect it is worth noting that certain aspects of osteopathic diagnosis have bioenergetic goals, similar to Tibetan medicine. Moreover some homoeopaths and medical herbalists do use subjective and intuitive methods of diagnosis, such as iridology and radiesthesia/radionics, although these are not generally accepted procedures.

Apparently by chance – or at least by some strange coincidence – it will be seen, as the contents of this section are progressively considered, that certain patterns of threes and fives and sometimes sevens, relevant to various classifications and categories, crop up with monotonous regularity. This applies particularly to what cycles by means of electronic instrumentation. Kirlian also evolved a special photographic technique to objectivize these. Both Burr and Kirlian discovered that they could predict illness before the appearance of any symptoms. Burr's conclusion was that the L Field is the organizing principle behind the physical structures. Jens Jerndal states:

> Impulses generated within this energy field are translated into chemical language by the endocrine glands, notably the pineal and pituitary. Chemical instruction from the glands are in their turn transformed into physiological building, decomposition or elimination processes that become visible as physical forms, shaping or disintegrating. This means that the only level of treatment which cannot be overruled is of the L-field itself, which is a vibrating, that is a wave-producing, energy structure. Characteristic of such a structure is its ability to resonate, to pick up certain vibratory characteristics from waves produced by other structures.
>
> The L-field can be influenced by many different agents, but they all have one thing in common: they are or produce radiation which has an effect on the L-field by way of resonance or interference, thus intensifying or disturbing its own natural wave-pattern. Among these agents we have cosmic influences, such as the energies generated by the movement of the planets, electric charges of the air, such as positively charged ions, musical notes (which are specific wavelengths of sound), colours (which are specific wavelengths of light), and all kinds of radiation such as X-rays. Radionics is entirely based on this level and is trying to codify this knowledge into a manageable technique. At the same time radionics is founded on the holographic principle of the universe, which means that each of the parts of a whole contains the complete picture of the whole, a principle which is also visible at the cell level, where each cell carries the DNA molecule bearing the genetic programme of the entire organism.
>
> Apparently homoeopathy also works on the L-field level, and that would explain the effect of the extremely small doses of the active substances. Acupuncture also works definitely on the L-field level, although the mechanism is not yet understood. Pulse diagnosis in acupuncture, as is known, can foretell faults in the energy structure not yet manifested in physical symptoms, just as Burr and Kirlian could with their respective methods.[4]

Rene Dubos, in the same decade, was also challenging with his book *The Mirage of Health*.[5] Contemporarily there is the monumental contribution of Fritjof Capra – his book *The Turning Point*[6] is an excellent example. In view of the two philosophical extremes of materialism and vitalism, von Bertalanfy pioneered the 'Systems Theory' in his book *Problems of Life*[7] some forty years ago, which from a Western scientific point of view emphasizes that living organisms depend basically on their 'inherent motility' for their functioning and not on any outside source of energy in an entity sense, e.g. *vis* Medicatrix Naturae, other than the all-pervasive cosmo-physical energies that express themselves through the basic warp and weft of the structures in terms of the Five Elements.

Let us continue to listen to what Jens Jerndal[8] and others have to say today:

> I imagine many readers will be familiar with the concept of chakras. These are centres in our energy fields, kinds of transformer stations for our vital energy, and they seem to be intimately linked with the glands. The glandular system is built up as a hierarchy with the pineal and pituitary glands at the top. Untill quite recently Western medical science knew practically nothing about the pineal gland, and the pituitary gland was also very little understood. On the whole this is still true. In the last two decades, however, highly significant discoveries have been made that open the way to a rational scientific explanation of some important and useful experiences made by astrologers and mediums that hitherto have been discarded by science as nonsensical fantasy.
>
> Among the few things we do know about the pineal gland are the following. Together with the pituitary and the hypothalamus, the pineal gland directs, via the hormones it produces, the activities of other glands. So, for instance, the pineal gland gives signals to the reproductive system, and it is the pineal gland which sets a child's birth in motion by producing a hormone that makes the womb contract and expel the baby.
>
> Also, the pineal gland is sensitive to ultra-violet radiation, that is, waves emitted by the sun. When there is no light, the

pineal gland produces a hormone called melatonin, which inhibits sexual activity and fertility. When there is light, however, the pineal gland produces another hormone called seratonin, which curbs melatonin production and stimulates sexual drive and fertility. The transformation of melatonin into seratonin or vice versa is performed with the help of ions of iron. From these established scientific facts, two observations are of prime importance for alternative medicine. The first is that the gland reacts to electromagnetic vibrations of a certain wavelength. If one gland reacts to one type of electromagnetic wave, then it is no longer superstitious nonsense to assume that the same gland – or other glands – may react also to other electromagnetic wavelengths. The second observation is that metal ions participate in the production of the hormones which actually direct the physiological processes of the body and thus indirectly run the whole show including metabolism, growth, regeneration of cells, functioning of the various organs and so on. In the case of melatonin it is iron, but there are excellent reasons to assume that other metals, notably magnesium, copper, mercury, lead, and zinc along with several others, play just as important a role for the glandular chemistry of the body. And there is now rapidly expanding awareness in modern Western medicine of the importance of minerals to health, even if we have not begun to understand the complexity of the matter.

This leads us to look at some sensational research, performed first on the initiative of Rudolf Steiner by Mrs L. Kolisko nearly sixty years ago and since then repeated many times, the latest to my knowledge by the English chemist Nick Kollerstrom. This research shows in as scientific way as anyone can demand how metal ions react to planetary vibration, and not only that, but how each of them is sensitive only to the planet with which astrological tradition has always connected them. These experiments show that lead ions react to Saturn, iron to Mars and silver to the moon. So to sum up, we have glands sensitive to electromagnetic vibrations, like waves from the sun and planets. These glands use metal ions in order to produce the hormones through which they govern chemically the functions of the organism. These metal ions have also been proved to react to the vibrations of certain planets.

In view of the knowledge thus gained it seems reasonable to hypothesize that the metals, with their special magnetic and electric properties, act as translators of the vital cosmic energies into the chemical language of the body. Moreover, the Swedish acupuncturist Dr Erik Bergström discovered that his acupuncture treatment did not work as it should in patients with serious mineral deficiencies.

On the other hand, my eminent friend Dr Lars-Olaf Berglöf in Stockholm found another reason why treatment sometimes does not have the expected effect. Upon closer observation, that unsuccessful treatment turned out to be linked with certain mental attitudes rooted in the unconscious, or in situations of emotional stress, which caused imbalances or faults in the energy field. As long as the emotional or mental stress persisted, the illness would not respond to treatment, or would recur after a short time. Dr Berglöf found that a way to cure this kind of patient was a course in mind control. The patient was taught to relax and dissolve the emotionally conditioned block, or strain, by positive reprogramming of his or her reflexes on an unconscious level. Once this was achieved, the illness often disappeared itself, as the energy resumed a free and balanced flow. And if the illness did not recede spontaneously, the patient would at least be receptive to the treatment, which would now be effective and give the expected result.

Glen Rein[9] takes up a similar theme regarding the importance of electro-magnetic fields in relation to psychic healing; and quotes recent experiments showing that electro-magnetic fields 'can carry biological information between two living systems separated by short distances'. On the question of healing at a distance he provides the following information which is extremely pertinent to our subject.

In the light of the newly discovered quantum mechanical properties of biological systems, where the collagen molecule has been shown to have piezoelectric properties, it is plausible that Bearden's theory can be extended to living tissues. Furthermore, since it is known that crystals in the pineal gland of the brain are composed of collagenous type molecules, these crystalline structures may be able to act as scalar interferometers. Thus, it is conceivable that during unusual brain activity associated with the healing state, acoustic energy generated by the specific neuronal firing patterns could generate enough pressure to cause the crystals in the pineal gland to emit scalar waves. These scalar waves could then couple with any of the myriad different EM (or other) energies likely to be emitted during healing, thereby generating triplet waves which could cause a unique biological response in the person being healed. Alternatively, the triplet waves could be used to carry the unique healing signal associated with the scalar waves over long distances. When the triplet waves arrive at the person being healed, they become decoupled and the original scalar wave causes the actual healing by coupling with the subject's own EM field. In this way a certain amount of healing specificity can be generated, since the healer's scalar wave will only couple with the healer's EM field if it is abnormal in such a way as to require the healer's specific scalar wave to cure it. Thus, in addition to offering a scientific explanation for distant healing, this new hypothesis also explains how psychic healing energy can contain a unique type of energy, the scalar wave, which although basically EM in nature would not be detectable by conventional EM detectors. It is the author's opinion that during psychic healing three types of energy are radiated:

(1) conventional EM/acoustic energy fields with unique healing properties, by virtue of their specific physical properties determined by their frequency, intensity, polarisation, coherence and degree of modulation;

(2) scalar waves; and

(3) triplet waves.

Each of these types of radiation is likely to have its own biological effects by modulating the healer's own endogenous EM field which, if diseased, will have a particular affinity for, and resonant interaction with, the healing radiation emitted by the healer. When the EM field is healed, the physical-chemical manifestations of disease will subsequently revert to a normal condition.

A Comparison of Western and Tibetan Medical Thought

Bridging the gap

What is the significance of this up-to-date Western scientific research to our attempts to bridge the gap between Western and Tibetan medical thinking? Two instances immediately come to mind:

(a) the ritual healing aspect of the latter, the intoning of mantras for various reasons, including the preparation of medicines, and

(b) the strange phenomenon of the 'family pulse' hitherto inexplicable by Western terms of logic.

When someone is too sick to travel to see the doctor, providing that the head of the family comes instead, the imbalances in the humours of the sick patient can be read on the relative's pulses. Similar prognostications can be made at a distance with the 'guest', 'enemy' and 'friend' pulses. At the pineal-gland ('third eye') level? It's fascinating food for thought.

Going back some forty years, J.E.R. McDonagh, FRCS, a prolific writer, was making very revolutionary statements in terms of his central theme, *The Universe through Medicine* (the title of his principal book).[10] All matter is a condensation of cosmic energy, he claimed, which he called 'Activity', the process evolving in a spiral sense through six cycles:

Pre-colloidal half of the spiral – exhibits no independence	1. Subatomic – involving the proton and neutron.
	2. Atomic – the elements are formed, metals, non-metals and inert gases.
	3. Crystalline – carbon being particularly relevant as the basis of all organic structures.
nascent independence	4. Colloid – the evolution of protein which allows the hitherto unique functions of the first three states to combine.

| beginnings of independence | 5. Vegetable – Protein – which differentiates the various species of the vegetable kingdom. |
| independence | 6. Animal – Protein – which forms the tissues and organs. |

Man, says McDonagh, is the final product, exhibiting complete independence.

'Activity' describes a double-cycle through the three sub-divisions of protein, the radiator, the attractor and storer portions. Consequently protein:

(a) pulsates, there is alternate rhythmic expansion and contraction, and

(b) in the process exhibits three functions: radiation, attraction and storage.

According to McDonagh, 'Activity' is able to describe these cycles by virtue of what he calls 'climate', or varying high-energy rays (he mentions cosmic rays), which continually penetrate every product, to varying depths and thus releases 'Activity'.

There is only one disease (hence the *Unitary Theory of Disease*) – all 'diseases' are merely aspects of imbalance or aberration manifest in the blood protein. The main aberration is an over-expansion or over-contraction of the whole, or of any of its parts, which may manifest either as acute, sub-acute, chronic, morbid inflammatory conditions, and cancer. As to which organs and tissues become involved, the nature of the symptoms will depend on which portions of the blood protein are involved in the imbalance. Figure 3 illustrates this point.

Cure, or a return to normality, can only come about when the imbalance in the blood protein has been restored. In the Nature of Disease Institute, McDonagh employed natural therapeutic methods principally as a means of restoring the balance of the blood protein: wholefood dietetics, colonic-irrigation, osteopathy to normalize viscero-somatic 'lesions' (with the Alexander Technique in order to maintain the corrections made), auto vaccines and various hormonal preparations. His approach to health and disease, both in terms of the nature of disease, its causation and

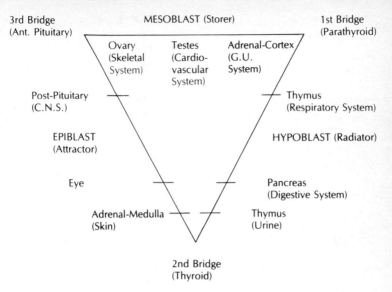

3rd Bridge
(Ant. Pituitary)

MESOBLAST (Storer)

1st Bridge
(Parathyroid)

Ovary
(Skeletal
System)

Testes
(Cardio-
vascular
System)

Adrenal-Cortex
(G.U.
System)

Post-Pituitary
(C.N.S.)

Thymus
(Respiratory System)

EPIBLAST
(Attractor)

HYPOBLAST (Radiator)

Eye

Pancreas
(Digestive System)

Adrenal-Medulla
(Skin)

Thymus
(Urine)

2nd Bridge
(Thyroid)

Figure 3 *Diagrammatic representation of blood protein (McDonagh's Triangle)*

prevention, plus the restoration of health, was totally holistic and ultimately bioenergetic.

It takes very little imagination to recognize the parallels in theory and practice between that of Tibetan medicine and McDonagh's unique Western conceptual model. Concerning the latter, Dr Laurence and others found medical dowsing to be eminently suitable as a vehicle for putting it into clinical practice.

J.E.R. McDonagh, FRCS, considered by many to be one of the greatest independent and original minds in medical research in this century, was mostly ignored by his medical colleagues during his most active and productive period, and both the man and his work are now virtually forgotten. At least he was not persecuted like his other striking contemporary, Wilhelm Reich.

I remember first hearing about McDonagh during the early 1950s from a visiting American osteopath, who spoke warmly about his research and its importance to osteopathic medicine. Later on I read an article in a medical Radiesthesia journal, 'Radiesthesia IV',[11] by Dr George Laurence, who was one of the great pioneers in this country of what is now called 'Bio-energetics'.

McDonagh was both a prolific writer and a highly erudite scientist. Therefore, for the less academically instructed, his books are extremely difficult to read. Both George Laurence and Aubrey Westlake have produced very readable précis, which are certainly worthy of further study. Of all of McDonagh's works, I personally found *The Nature of Disease Up to Date* (1946) and *The Universe in the Making* (1948), to be both reasonably understandable and invaluable in my quest for knowledge and understanding of holistic medicine and healing. This has led me ultimately to the study of Tibetan medicine.

It is timely to briefly mention Dr H. Laborit,[12] and the study that he has made in relation to body-reaction mechanisms in terms of shock and/or stress, by which the physical body maintains homeostasis. In order to do this, the organism functions in terms of oscillating phases around the point of equilibrium. This oscillating movement explains the phase of stress and counter-stress found in the alarm reaction of Selye, with its primary sympathetic phase which is subsequently followed by a stage of vagotonia, which is, incidentally, typical of a disease of traumatic origin. This constant attempt to maintain equilibrium in terms of opposite phases of function applies equally to biocatalysis, thus explaining the opposite and successive functions of the bio-catalysts, e.g. calcium and potassium, histamine, acetylcholine, adrenalin, the gluco and minuralo-corticoids, etc., in which one or other synergetic groups become alternatively predominant in each succeeding phase. This, Laborit has called 'the oscillating post-stress reaction' (OPSR). He wrote:

The harmonious O.P.S.R. gradually fades out in terms of time and the amplitude of each oscillating phase and its duration is directly related to the reactional possibility of the organism. The O.P.S.R. which is not harmonious or successful, fails to completely follow through in terms of the swinging phases, and each phase is cut short to the detriment of the other, e.g. an anabolic or vagotonic phase that is prematurely aborted in favour of the sympathetic or catabolic phase. Unless one takes this into consideration, all accumulated knowledge in terms of chemical mediation, electrolyte metabolism, the functions of different hormones and particularly ACTH, the gluco-corticoids, the mineral corticoids, and the androgens is difficult to understand. Interpreted in this way one sees the inter-relation of either synergetic or contrary actions of different ergones, vaso-motor phenomena, the different metabolic functions, the functions of the reticulo-endothelial system, basic tissue reactions etc.

The O.P.S.R. is described according to its different reactional phases:

1. The immediate phase of disturbed equilibrium; the balance existing between the organism and its environment is broken with two eventual possibilities –

   (a) If the balance between the organism and its environment passes a certain threshold the classical signs of shock will appear.

   (b) If on the other hand the stressors are of a less severe order, they may cause no more than mild transient disturbances or no symptoms may appear at all. If, however, they are constantly repeated they may present a considerable danger, for the very reason that oscillating reactions of a feeble but repetitive amplitude are liable to provoke, over a long period of time, morbid and chronic symptoms (the adaptation diseases of Selye).

2. The phase of neuro-vegetative reaction: if the stress factors are not sufficient to overwhelm the organism the first line of defence is by means of nerve reflexes and this reaction is characterised by a frank discharge of adrenalin: this reaction is essentially catabolic.

   If this self-defence should prove efficacious, a new and temporary state of equilibrium appears which is opposite to the preceding one, and this too tends to resolve in relation to the basic point of equilibrium. The different factors which characterise phase number one are generally reversed during the phase of neuro-vegetative reaction. A neuro-endocrine reaction may also enter the picture at this stage, a reaction which is also catabolic. If the nerve reflex defence therefore proves inadequate, the neuro-endocrine system of defence comes into play, and this stage may last during four or five days.

3. Anabolic stage. An organism in a state of disequilibrium may be obliged to bring into play an additional mechanism of self-defence in order to regain its balance. This however does not always occur immediately and the previous reaction or stage of disequilibrium may be reversed. However, the reaction engendered by the original stress factor continues to reduce progressively, and becomes more diffused, and the duration of this new and ultimate phase of disequilibrium usually lasts eight to ten days; this is the vagotonic crisis which usually appears on the 4th or 5th day. All the symptoms which appear depend upon a histamo-cholinergic mechanism. However, if histamine and acetylcholine possess doubtful vaso-motor properties, they do exert a positive biological and metabolic influence. They encourage inflammation, hyperaemia, the mobilization of reticulocytes, and their role in scar formation and tissue healing appears to be fundamental. From a neuro-endocrine point of view, during this period the mineral-corticoids are predominant, with their beneficial effect on tissue granulation. This applies also to the androgens whose anabolic properties are well known, as is that of somatrophin. It would seem that this vagal phase is the complementary reaction to the inverse and preceding phase of disequilibrium which is adreno-catabolic, and which is itself reactive to the initial stress. During this phase any histo-physio-pathology that is present during the catabolic phase resolves. One sees that in effect the anabolic phase, which is the longest, finally predominates in long-term stress of average intensity. The harmonious reaction that we have just described is such as will occur in the average healthy organism, which has been able to contain its reaction within the purview of homeostasis.

4. On the contrary one can have disharmonious reaction which outlives its usefulness, with pathological consequences (maladaptation). This is liable to occur when the stress factors are sufficiently intense and therefore able to overwhelm the reactional ability of the organism. This is

particularly so if the stress factors are sufficiently frank and brutal. For instance a spectacular primary defence reaction to stress may well engender a chaotic secondary catabolic phase, which is terminal.

Laborit's scientific findings are thus found to substantiate the Buddhist and Tibetan medical philosophical tenets, as expressed by Gyatso Tshering and Lama Govinda.

Mind over Matter

In Chapter 15 some interesting and convincing improvements in health by sufferers from hypertension are mentioned, in respect of some controlled clinical trials, involving Buddhist meditation techniques. The following Report also provides more Western scientific proof of 'mind over matter' so to speak. In *Nature* vol. 295, 21 January 1983:

> Since meditative practices are associated with changes that are consistent with decreased activity of the sympathetic nervous system, it is conceivable that measurable body temperature changes accompany advanced meditative states. With the help of H.H. the Dalai Lama, we have investigated such a possibility on three practitioners of the advanced Tibetan Buddhist meditational practice known as g Tum-mo (heat) yoga living in Upper Dharamsala, India. We report here that in a study performed there in February 1981, we found that these subjects exhibited the capacity to increase the temperature of their fingers and toes by as much as $8.3°C$.
>
> g Tum-mo yoga is a form of meditation which allegedly allows its practitioners to alter body temperature. Previously, only subjective descriptions of this phenomenon existed: 'The neophytes sit on the ground, cross-legged and naked. Sheets are dipped in icy water, each man wraps himself in one of them and must dry it on his body. As soon as the sheet has become dry, it is again dipped in the water and placed on the novice's body to be dried as before. The operation goes on in that way until daybreak. Then he who has dried the largest number of sheets is declared the winner of the competition'.

During the practice of g Tum-mo yoga, 'prāna' (literally, 'wind' or 'air') is withdrawn from the scattered condition of normal consciousness and is made to enter into the 'central channel' inside the body. Then, through the alleged dissolution of these winds in the central channel, the 'internal heat' is ignited. The physiological changes are, therefore, a by-product of a religious practice.

Each of the three monks in the present investigation had spent more than 6 years practising g Tum-mo daily and had lived most of the past 10 years in near-isolation in unheated, uninsulated stone huts – 4 × 7 m. The floors were earthen and the roofs made of large slate slabs or flattened tin cans. The huts were in isolated locales in the foothills of the Himalayan Mountains at altitudes of 1,800–2,000 m, outside the town of Upper Dharamsala. The first two subjects were studied in their hermitages while the third was studied in a hotel room in Upper Dharamsala. Each participated in the investigation after being asked to do so by H.H. the Dalai Lama. Verbal informed consent was obtained from the three subjects through our translator (Jeffrey Hopkins).

The subjects in the current experiment exhibited a greater capacity to warm fingers than has been previously recorded during hypnosis and after biofeedback training. Although it is possible that the practitioners had learned to increase their metabolism to produce more body heat, this seems unlikely. Even though they were all lean, the monks claimed not to require more than a 'normal' amount of food. Furthermore, their resting heart rates were within normal limits. The most likely mechanism to account for the increase in finger and toe temperature is vasodilation. Although no direct measurements of peripheral blood flow were made, others have calculated that during the simple meditative process of transcendental meditation, there is a 44% increase in nonhepatic, nonrenal blood flow and they hypothesized an increase in skin or cerebral blood flow or both.

g Tum-mo is one of the six Doctrines of Naropa, the great Indian Tantric Mahasiddha, some of whose teachings are discussed further on by Herbert Guenther in a different context (see Chapter 15).

Anatomy and Physiology

In Table 7 some limited correlation of the Western sciences of anatomy and physiology with the Three Humours is attempted, taking the musculo-skeletal and nervous system, central and autonomic, as a starting-point.

Table 7 An approximate correlation of the Western science of anatomy and physiology with the Three Humours

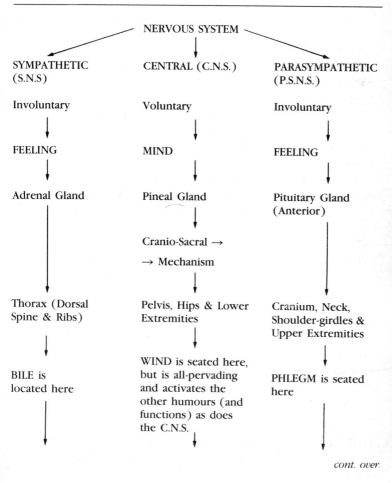

SYMPATHETIC (S.N.S)	NERVOUS SYSTEM CENTRAL (C.N.S.)	PARASYMPATHETIC (P.S.N.S.)
Involuntary	Voluntary	Involuntary
FEELING	MIND	FEELING
Adrenal Gland	Pineal Gland	Pituitary Gland (Anterior)
	Cranio-Sacral → → Mechanism	
Thorax (Dorsal Spine & Ribs)	Pelvis, Hips & Lower Extremities	Cranium, Neck, Shoulder-girdles & Upper Extremities
BILE is located here	WIND is seated here, but is all-pervading and activates the other humours (and functions) as does the C.N.S.	PHLEGM is seated here

cont. over.

Table 7 *cont.*

SYMPATHETIC (S.N.S.)	CENTRAL (C.N.S.)	PARASYMPATHETIC (P.S.N.S.)
Energy of Transformation (Carrier function)	Energy of the Mind and of the Cell	Energy of Flesh and Matter
Katabolism	Metabolism	Anabolism
Calcium Cholesterin H Ions – Adrenalin		Potassium Lecithin OH Ions – Cholin
Dehydration	Normal Fluid-Balance	Hydration
Function of Contraction		Function of Expansion
Cardio-vascular System	Voluntary functions of all systems i.e. Motor, Sensory & Trophic	Lymphatic System
ECTOMORPH (Sheldon)	MESOMORPH (Sheldon)	ENDOMORPH (Sheldon)
RADIATOR-MAN (McDonagh)	STORER-MAN (McDonagh)	ATTRACTOR-MAN (McDonagh)
Activity and Positive feeling-tone, but with Anxiety and Extroversion	Will, thinking, perception Aggressive Anxiety expressing itself as Extroversion	Passivity and Negative feeling-tone, Hysteria, Introversion

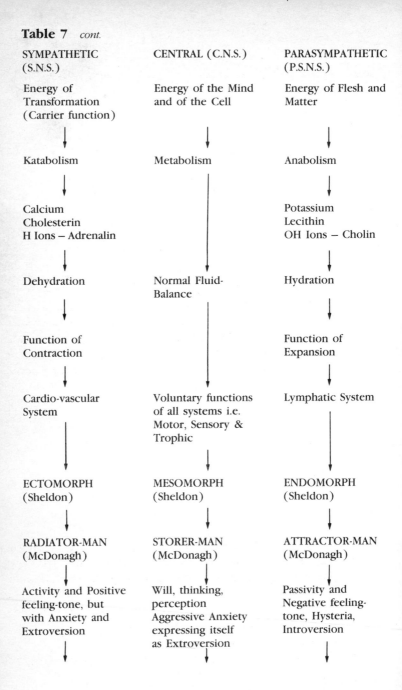

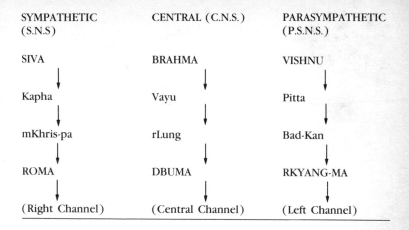

SYMPATHETIC (S.N.S)	CENTRAL (C.N.S.)	PARASYMPATHETIC (P.S.N.S.)
SIVA	BRAHMA	VISHNU
↓	↓	↓
Kapha	Vayu	Pitta
↓	↓	↓
mKhris-pa	rLung	Bad-Kan
↓	↓	↓
ROMA	DBUMA	RKYANG-MA
↓	↓	↓
(Right Channel)	(Central Channel)	(Left Channel)

The correlations shown in Table 7 are not static and syllogistic as a product of linear thinking. They reflect rather the steady state of relative dynamism (homeostasis). For example, passivity or inactivity has no substantive quality in itself. It becomes 'something' only in the absence of activity. This is rather in the Taoist sense that Yin is either merely an absence of Yang, or relatively there is less Yin if there is more Yang and vice versa. Once again whether it be in terms of any of the three groupings above, it's always a question of relative equilibrium between all three aspects of the 'whole', which are indivisible and inter-dependent.

Conclusions

A further summary of 'thought-bridges' will be found on p. 245. Meantime in résumé it can be said that:

(a) In 'holistic' medical terms, there appears to be a strong basis for a common understanding of clinical problems and procedures, between practitioners, of either Tibetan or Western medicine.
(b) A basic acknowledgment of either the same or, in some instances, similar, causative factors in disease, both in the immediate and longer-term future.
(c) Similarly with the psycho-somatic, functional, physio-

pathological basis of disease as expressed by imbalances of the three humours. The pathologies and degenerations take their rightful place of course.

(d) There is no disagreement as to the role of bio-energy, for want of a better term, englobing all forms of life-energy and the particular relevance of electro-magnetic fields and energies (and the pineal gland) in health and disease, and that different energies, from the most refined to the most crude, can affect each other for better or for worse.

(e) Nor as to the importance of 'patterns' and 'biorhythms' in health and disease.

(f) The Tantric 'inherent motility' principle stands in the middle of the extremes of the mechanistic and vitalistic views of life − both being equally dogmatic. Tibetan medicine, as with all other holistic medicines, relates directly with the contemporary Western 'Systems Theory'.

(g) Glen Rein's scientific hypothesis, concerning diagnostic and healing phenomena at a distance is extremely relevant.

(h) The Buddhist view that all is ultimately Mind, which in its pure and pristine state is 'The Adibuddha Kuntuzangpo who is and represents knowledge which is inseparable from the universal foundation, a plenum of all-pervasive, primal space', is the theme, unconscious or not, of J.E.R. McDonagh, FRCS, in his explanation of the *Universe through Medicine*. Also the scientific appraisal of the physiological changes occurring during g Tum-mo Yoga − mind over matter.

Tibetan medicine may well be part of an emergent historical cluster, in terms of the almost virtual 'explosion' in the West of holistic medicine. Of course it is another conceptual model, as indeed are all other systems of medicine. But there again, differing conceptual models, in whatever field of human activity, result from differing ways of looking at the world and existence generally.

In Mahayana Buddhist terms the different conceptual models of samsara are 'forms' which are conditioned by race, culture, religion, and which emerge from the Void, firstly as projection of the mind, which in their turn materialize into what Marxists delight in calling 'objective reality'.

As Dr Tashigang so delightfully put it, when we recently met in Delhi, in explaining the common factors and similarities between different systems of medicine in different cultures – 'One cooks the same chicken in a variety of different ways, according to country, culture and taste, but it's still the same chicken'.

This of course tallies perfectly with what His Holiness the Dalai Lama has said, and continues to re-affirm:

> All systems of medicine have their weak and strong points. It is desirable therefore, that there should be an open-minded approach, and active co-operation between all medicines, so as to allow the maximum benefit for everyone. Anything that we amongst others can do, to make better known by all possible means the particular benefits of Tibetan medicine is good.

In an introductory sense these are some of the generalities on which I have tried to 'build the bridge'. More explicit correlations and parallels will be found in the subsequent chapters, together with a final attempt at some kind of synthesis in the conclusions at the end.

A Brief Comparison of Tibetan and Chinese Medicine

First of all there are important philosophical differences between the two different medicines. The Yin/Yang concept of Chinese medicine is based on the Tao, whereas Buddha Dharma forms the basis of Tibetan medicine. While the Tao is primarily concerned with the 'search for immortality', Buddha Dharma stresses the impermanence of life and all compounded things. Indeed, according to Dzogchen there is ultimately no goal, object or perceiver, therefore there is no immortality as such and therefore, no search nor searcher. Moreover, the Yin/Yang concept is in itself a basic dualistic thinking system, the theory being based on the philosophical notion of two polar complements Yin and Yang, whereas, on the contrary, Buddha Dharma is essentially concerned with developing non-dualistic thinking.

Chinese and Tibetan medicine are therefore expressing philosophical opposites in their methodological approach to health and disease, although on the level of absolute truth, prana, rlung and ch'i are the same, the primordial all-pervading universal energy. Tibetan medicine expresses perfectly and cogently the idea and action relating to cause and effect, indeed finding the cause and attempting to at least eradicate or neutralize it (in which case this is achieved either by patient, practitioner or both together) and is of primary importance. Whereas dealing with the effect(s), is normally considered of secondary importance.

Chinese medicine, on the other hand, is not really so much concerned with the cause, as rather dealing with the effect, viz.: 'For the Chinese however, phenomena occur independently of an external act of creation, and there is no great need to search for a cause' (Ted J. Kaptchuk).[13]

Apart from such fundamental differences on the philosophical level, there is similarity on other levels, such as the pulses, the Five-Elements and mother/son, friend/foe relationships and the classification of organs, etc. For the purpose of comparison, as far as the pulse finger placements are concerned, please refer to Table 6, chapter 5 (p. 79). This gives the positions of the pulse according to the three traditions – the Ayurvedic, the Chinese and the Tibetan.

In conclusion:

Yin equates with bad-kan (Phlegm)
Yang equates with mkhris-pa (Bile)
Ch'i equates with rlung (Wind)

as similarly expressed in the terms 'Hot and Cold diseases'.

12

Western Herbal Medicine

Traditional and Contemporary Aspects

These aspects involve a study of the use of therapeutic plants and how their classical prescription may be adapted in terms of practising Tibetan medicine. The various systems of herbal medicine, i.e. the use of therapeutic plants and flora in the treatment of disease are common to all civilizations and cultures. With their roots and origins firmly in the past, many are nevertheless still flourishing.

The persistent theme of the first half of the twentieth century was 'it can't be any good unless it has been proven scientifically'. In view of this herbal medicine was forced, along with other heterodox therapies, to make every effort to conform to the dictates of science. Due, in the UK, to the efforts of Fred Fletcher-Hyde, Albert Priest, Albert Orbell, Fellows of the Medical Herbalists UK Institute in the last decade, names that spring easily to mind, plus more contemporary members such as Simon Mills, a truly scientific basis has been evolved for what is known as the physiomedical system of herbal medicine, a far cry from the traditional and empirical dispensations of the lady of the manor.

Incidentally in relation to our primary subject Tibetan medicine, similar research according to the scientific method is now being carried out by a Tibetan, Kelsang Rapten B. Sc. (Biochemistry) at the University of California, Irvine, USA.*

The history of Western herbal medicine is fascinating and

---

* 'gSorig', Series no. 3, 1981

149

mention of the lady of the manor was in no way meant to be in the pejorative. The works of Culpeper and Gerard are classics in terms of the practice of herbal medicine in the pre-scientific era, and are of great value. As Simon Mills[1] says, 'In every rural community since time began there were likely to be individuals, most often women ("wise-women") regarded as specialists in the art of using the healing plants'. One wonders in passing how many of them, when religious persecution was at its height in the UK for instance, were burnt at the stake as witches?

The Physiomedical System

The physiomedical system originated in the nineteenth century in North America as a result of a blend of European herbal practice, with its cultural origins in ancient Greek classicism, and the indigenous North American medicine. Principally associated with its development were such figureheads as Samuel Thomson, W. Beach, W.H. Cook, T.J. Lyle and J.M. Thurston.

Samuel Thomson (1769–1843), the pioneer of the physio-medical movement, in his book *New Guide to Health; or Botanic Family Physician* (Boston, 1835) makes the following statement, which from the point of view of Tibetan medicine is riveting – (I quote Simon Mills) –

> I found that all animal bodies were formed of four elements;
> the Earth and Water constitute the solid; and the Air and Fire
> (or Heat) are the cause of life and motion; that cold, or the
> lessening of the power of heat is the cause of all disease; that to
> restore heat to its natural state was the only way health could
> be produced, and that after restoring the natural heat, by
> clearing the system of all obstruction and causing a natural
> perspiration, the stomach would digest the food taken into it,
> and the heat (or nature) be enabled to hold her supremacy.

Apart from the over-riding importance stressed by Thomson of restoring heat and vital activity in order to reconstitute and maintain the life-processes, re-equilibration of the nervous system *in toto* must take place simultaneously in order to effect satisfactory homeostasis, i.e. the dynamic balance between anabolism (absorption and use of nutrition) and catabolism (elimination of the by-products of metabolism) and therefore health.

W.H. Cook added another dimension. To again quote Simon Mills —

> Cook saw biological life as a harmonious oscillation between activity and inactivity, with disease heralded by an excess at one functional level or other. He essentially saw herbal remedies as being able to correct excessive tensions (by 'relaxants') or excessive relaxation (states) – (by 'astringents'), while still retaining their overall enhancement of vitality.

Accordingly, the basic physiomedical principles, the three aspects of therapeutic objective, are in terms of balancing the physio-chemical processes of the body to:

1. Relax and warm (heat), both systemically and selectively.
2. Astringe and cool (calm down), both systemically and selectively.
3. Stimulate in terms of invigorating and increasing body vitality and tone generally, and directing energy specifically in a synergistic and supportive sense, to the local systemic/visceral/cellular influences of Relaxing and Astringing accordingly. *Of primordial importance*, the degree or quality of stimulation must never exceed the capacity of the organism to respond positively. Over-stimulation leads to further exhaustion and depletion, and of course increased imbalance.

Classically, J.M. Thurston emphasized the importance of vaso-motor regulation of the visceral functions via the vaso-motor system. Herbal medicines, in addition to being classified as relaxants, astringents and stimulants are listed as:

1. Vaso-stimulants
2. Vaso-relaxants
3. Vaso-dilators
4. Vaso-compressors
5. Vaso-tonics – which include alterative and tropho-restorative medicines.

Simon Mills mentions that, in the light of more recent physiological research, this hypothesis may have to be up-dated in order to provide a more contemporary explanation. This of course is equally true of all holistic medical systems whose roots lie in the pre-scientific age, where clinical interpretations were based solely on religious, philosophical, empirical and intuitive considerations. Such up-dating would certainly please the 'mechanists' and also those who seem to be more concerned with this particular modern form of ego-gratification, i.e. the obsession for being scientific, rather than being of assistance to the object of all medicinal care – *the patients*. In fact, these and every aspect of the sum total of all existing knowledge pertinent to *helping the patient* should be taken into consideration.

It is of interest, too, that Simon Mills mentions the Galenic tradition of classifying herbs into hot and cold, and points out that this is also inherent in Chinese medicine. Moreover he makes reference to Dr Yeshi Donden – Tibetan Master Physician – in the Bibliography to his article.

In conclusion, the physiomedical system may in simplistic terms be said to be based on this synthesis:

(a) The vitalist Five Element view as laid down by Thomson.
(b) The depurative and body detoxifying aspects as being fundamental in treatment, emetics, sweat-baths and diaphoretics playing a big part, emphasized by Beach.
(c) The localized tissue-reaction approach, i.e. specific remedies for specific organs and their diseases, the more symptomatic treatment aspect according to Lyle.
(d) The 'physiological' mode, i.e. of treating and re-balancing the body's functions through the autonomic, vaso-motor system, Thurston's contribution.[2]
(e) Herbal medicines are administered with a view to:
   1. relaxing and warming;
   2. astringing and cooling;
   3. stimulating – activating, energy-directing, sustaining and supporting. Consequently:
(f) The botanical agents contained in Materia Medica are classified as:

1. Relaxants
2. Astringents } both systemic and as organ specifics
3. Stimulants

plus the five vaso-motor propensies, with an additional category of Alteratives, Antiseptics, etc.

This basic thumb-nail picture may be said to constitute the physiomedical system of herbal medicine, as has been developed and maintained and is practised in the UK, principally by members of the National Institute of Medical Herbalists, and as taught in their associated School in Tunbridge Wells, Kent, England.

Holistic and Cosmological Aspects

The holistic and cosmological aspects of plant medicines are exemplified as follows:

(a) by the traditional practice of using preparations in various forms of either the whole plant itself or, singly, the intact whole parts, whereas allopathic medicine extracts the 'active-principle' – the alkaloids – and usually combines these with some chemical base.

(b) by the empirically (well-known for several centuries) qualities of certain herbs as having a curative effect on the mind and emotions as well as the soma, i.e. their action is psychosomatic in terms of the 'whole' person. Rue (Ruta graveolans) for madness and Mistletoe (Viscum album) for hysteria are just two that come to mind. Such plants and aspects have been the subject of considerable study and experiment, particularly in astrological terms, by the English herbalists Culpeper and Gerard.

and that:

(c) herbs, as with other vegetation, are the product through the nitrogen and carbon cycles of the inter-reaction of the Five Elements: Air, Fire (heat), Water, Earth and within the cosmos – Space.

(d) whole herbs can provide:

(1) Nutrition { including protein, carbohydrate, fat, minerals, vitamins, hormones, etc.
(2) the five Energies of the Five Elements
(3) specific therapeutic properties in terms of plant alkaloids — the 'active-principles'.

Correlations between Western and Tibetan Medicine

In attempting to relate the Tibetan medical viewpoint to the physiomedical system, let us consider the very simplistic (on the face of it) physiomedical formula as devised by Cook. As Simon Mills says:

> He (Cook) was convinced that each tissue manifested a tidal rhythm of alternating action and inaction (as seen most simply in the beat of the heart), and that this periodicity was an essential feature of biological life. We now know that he was perfectly correct in this assumption. He thus saw the health of each tissue, each cell, as being maintained by the smooth oscillation between activity and inactivity, neither one predominating. Disease he saw therefore as explicable in terms of the tissues concerned being either too active ('tensed') or too inactive ('relaxed') for healthy function, and the aim of herbal therapy therefore was to relax the overtense and 'astringe' the over-relaxed.

This can be expressed thus:

Tissues that are:
(a) Over-active and tense — require Relaxant medicines.
(b) Inactive and over-relaxed — require Astringent Contractant medicines.
(c) Depressed and low in vitality, i.e. tissue and systemic innervation — require stimulants.

The use of the word 'Contractant' is preferred by some physiomedicalists since, as applied to some botanical agents, the term 'Astringent' has a certain ambiguity. The physiological properties of Relaxants and Contractants connote a balancing-up action or movement on a horizontal plane, whereas Stimulants enhance vitality in the upward vertical plane. By the same token sedatives operate on the downward vertical plane.

In the physiomedical Materia Medica there are of course agents that stimulate and sedate (in the vertical plane) and others that relax and contract either generally or systematically, and others that act locally on specific organs and tissues. Moreover certain herbs stimulate in one sense and at the same time relax in another, etc., etc., according to the different tissues that are being influenced, e.g. the different tissues in the same organ. This is why matters are not as simplistic as they may appear on the surface.

In view of what is after all a very complex subject let us try nevertheless to equate Tibetan medical concepts with those of physiomedicalism. Assuming that tissues are over-tense either in terms of inflammation and/or hyperfunction, they are also usually *Hot*. The hyperfunction is horizontal and the *heat* aspect is vertical in an upward direction. Such a condition would correspond in Tibetan (or Chinese) medicine with what is generally called a Hot disease.

The same principle applies to tissues that are inactive and (over) relaxed either in terms of fluid stasis and/or hypofunction. The hypofunction is a horizontal manifestation, and the *cold* aspect is vertical in a downward direction. Such a condition would correspond in Tibetan (or Chinese) medicine with what is generally called a Cold disease. (In Tibetan medicine all pure Wind (rLung) diseases are neutral. In a similar way, within the autonomic nervous system the para-sympathetic and sympathetic aspects do not always identify entirely with the Yin and Yang principles (i.e. Hot and Cold) nor do the Hot and Cold diseases of Tibetan medicine entirely co-relate with the Physiomedical model.)

In Tibetan medicine there is a parallel with the duality mentioned above in relation to the actual botanical agents themselves, in terms of the clinical requirements of the disturbed organ or tissue itself, which may require general stimulation in one sense and specific relaxation in another. The parallel with Tibetan medicine is that it is seldom that one humour is involved on its own, indeed clinically there are often two involved or even all three at times (please refer to Chapter 4, p. 69).

Similarly with physiomedical prescribing. Contractants for example may be mixed wth Relaxants, i.e. addressed to different levels within the same system, organ or tissue, or the clinical problem may rather call for a general Stimulant or Relaxant like Capsicum minim or Lobelia inflater accordingly.

Generally this complex issue can be summed up as follows:

The Three Humours	mKhris-pa (Fire)	Hot diseases	tissues over-tense and hot; treated principally by Relaxants
	Bad-kan (Earth & Water)	Cold diseases	tissues over-relaxed and cold; treated principally by Contractants (Astringents)
	rLung (Air)	Neutral	treated by Stimulants combined either with Relaxants or Astringents accordingly

All are categorized in terms of the Five Energies of the Five Elements and the five related aspects of vaso-motion plus the inclusion of other classes of botanical agents, such as alteratives, anti-septics, etc., according to the clinical requirements for the individual patient.

Materia Medica

Information is available in the appropriate literature and from the pharmaceutical houses that supply either crude herbs, fluid-extracts, tinctures or tablets, regarding the wide range of herbs and herbal medicines available. While many of these are very similar to those used in classical Tibetan medicine, it must be stipulated that *only* crude herbs as such are actually identical. Albert and Priest's book contains a very comprehensive botanic materia medica.[3]

Conclusions

In view of the difficulty of procuring and maintaining supplies of Tibetan medicines at the moment, qualified physiomedical practitioners need have no great problem in adapting their own system and philosophy to that of Tibetan medicine, should they so desire. Obviously this would not be the same, since the Tibetan Materia Medica uses other substances from nature apart from plants. There is a point worth mentioning however: it has been stressed for example that the properties of medicinal plants gathered on the Tibetan side of the Himalayas are not necessarily the same as the identical plants found on the Indian side, for obvious reasons. The indigenous plants are said to be more efficacious, which is understandable from a geographical/climatic point-of-view.

It is a generally held view in the West that indigenous foods and plant medicines are superior for diet and medicinal usage. The hypothesis is – perhaps medicines made from plants indigenous to the UK and Europe may be more suitable and effective in those countries than those imported from India and/or Tibet? Also, perhaps there are ethnic differences which may have a bearing? Barry Clark strongly disagrees. Anyway it's food for thought.

In the West it should be noted that plant medicines prepared according to Rudolf Steiner principles accord very closely to the Tibetan procedures, i.e. the cosmological considerations are taken into account, particularly with their gathering.

13

Homoeopathy

How Homoeopathy can be adapted within the Philosophy of Tibetan Medicine

Homoeopathy as a method of medical treatment was founded by Samuel Christian Hahnemann, a doctor born in Saxony in Germany in 1755. The fundamental law of cure upon which all homoeopathic prescribing is based is known as the 'Law of Similars' – *similia similibus curentur*.[1] Hahnemann discovered purely by chance that Cinchona Bark (from which quinine is derived) which was then used to treat malaria, when given in material dosage produced in healthy subjects symptoms similar to those of malaria itself. Hahnemann experimented both on himself and volunteers with a number of other therapeutic substances in use at the time, and found similarly. The use of Belladonna for Scarlet Fever is another well-quoted case in point. These correspondences he called 'provings' and there are now some three thousand of these in the modern homoeopathic Materia Medica. Basically, the remedies are given in very minimal dosage to sick persons whose symptoms correspond to those that would be provoked by the drug if given to healthy persons. Different diseases produce typical symptom-complexes, the totality of which constitutes the 'disease-picture'. The symptom-complex which a normally therapeutic substance could cause when a healthy person ingests a substantial dose is known as the 'drug-picture'. When the 'drug-picture' matches the 'disease picture', the remedy responsible for the former cancels out and/or annuls the 'disease picture'. The more accurately this can be done, the better the results are likely to be. Such a specific remedy is known as the 'simillimum'.

Charles Wheeler, MD[2] in 1920 explained the action of homoeopathic medicines as follows:

> Disease is ultimately an affair of the reactions of protoplasm, and in the response of protoplasm to stimuli we should find, if anywhere, material for generalisations upon disease and treatment. Now these responses of protoplasm have been well investigated, and appear to follow a constant rule generally summarised as Arndt's Law. The simple statement of this rule is that small stimuli encourage life activity, medium to strong stimuli tend to impede it, and very strong stimuli to stop or destroy it. (Thus strong solutions of arsenious acid will destroy the yeast cell, less strong impede its fermentative activity, but very dilute solutions will encourage its activity, at any rate for a time.)
>
> Considering only the behaviour of protoplasm, we should be led to argue that since in disease the cells specially attacked are the cells specially in need of a stimulus (since their life activities are threatened), that stimulus will be found in a small dose of the agent which in large dose can damage or destroy precisely these particular cells. How can the special relationships of drugs to cells be known? How but by a testing of drugs upon the healthy? Drugs given to persons in health will influence certain cells and tissues according to their individual 'affinities': when by symptoms thus produced we know that a drug can damage this or that set of cells, then we can use a small dose of the same drug to stimulate the same set of cells if oppressed by disease. In other words, the responses of protoplasm to stimuli would justify the recommendations:
>
> a) When treating disease, look for a drug which has produced similar symptoms on the healthy, for only thus can there be any confidence that it will influence the tissues affected.
> b) Give a small dose.

The special way of preparing the actual medicines in minimal dosage is discussed further on.

Radionic practitioners who prescribe homoeopathic remedies obviously take a less material view. Based rather on 'energetic' considerations, for them every substance has its own particular wave-length or vibrational pattern which is called a 'standing-wave'. The homoeopathic healing phenomenon, it is believed, occurs when the remedy concerned has the same 'standing-wave' as the disease.

To summarize, there are three important laws relative to the practice of homoeopathy, the two already mentioned – the 'Law of Similars' and Arndt's Law – plus Hering's Law, which says that 'healing takes place from above downwards and from within outwards'. These three laws constitute the basis of clinical homoeopathic medicine.

In Chapter 3 it was mentioned that the totality of all life processes both within living organisms and in the external environment, and in the relationship between the two, is an expression of the five cosmo-physical energies which again manifest as the Five Elements, Air, Water, Fire, Earth and Space. Moreover it was pointed out that these elements are not just material, but have their own inherent energy-function qualities. Whether it be the medicines prescribed or the body/mind organism treated, all is composed, as is indeed is everything in the universe, of the five cosmo-physical energies or elements.

The principle of 'like cures like', the fundamental basis of classical homoeopathy, is a permanent anathema to mechanistically-minded persons who cannot possibly conceive, understand or indeed accept the idea that any other qualities exist in medicinal substances, other than the gross physiochemical. Yet here is the answer, the total answer in fact to the anathema – all medicines in the final analysis are composed of the same Five Elements and, equally, so are all living organisms, be they healthy or diseased.

How medicines may be conceived, prepared and administered, and with what conceptual purpose is another matter. Dualistic thinking allows for difference, diversity and fragmentation both in concept, intent and practical application. Allopathic medicine splits up naturally occurring substances into their component parts, as well as synthesizing others artificially, extracting their 'active principles' which are then laboratory tested in isolation from the greater cosmo-physical context. This is done in order to establish their efficacy in modifying usually in an alterative sense certain groups of symptoms ('specific diseases') on the principle of cure by opposites. This also permits 'biological standardization', a very necessary procedure when dealing commonly with such varieties and combinations of the Five Elements, many of the side-effects of which are potentially more upsetting than the often transient symptomatic relief afforded by the drug at the time.

This is not an emotional or irresponsible attack on the allopathic system of medicine, quite the contrary. Indeed what is being said about the problem of iatrogenesis is a pre-occupying source of worry to more and more allopathically trained, practising physicians.

Homoeopathy, as conceived and founded as a school of thought and medical practice by Samuel Hahnemann about three centuries ago, was a revolt in a polar-opposite sense against the then exceedingly crude allopathic-system, with its highly dangerous and toxic remedies, i.e. as it was practised before the scientific basis of modern medicine was established.

Hahnemann's discoveries regarding cure by similars, the minimal dose, and the clinical fact that the potency of remedial substances increases in direct proportion to their material make-up being progressively reduced (and one assumes their energy content being equally increased), was revolutionary. This qualitative change is effected by a process initiated by Hahnemann, called Trituration. By syllogistic reasoning the increased potency of a remedy equals the increase in its energy aspect or content, the two being synonymous. Low potencies of remedies contain a mixture of both physiochemical content and the potentized energy of the substance.

High-potencies, especially when they are very high, contain nothing more than pure energy or, in a Tibetan medicinal term, the 'pure essence' of the remedy. This understandably explains why analyses by normal laboratory analytical procedures find that the pills contain nothing more than the sugar of milk vehicle of which they are materially composed. Boyd[3] and co-workers in Glasgow, however, were able to establish effective means of demonstrating that homoeopathic medicines do contain what they are supposed to contain.

Concerning homoeopathy in the UK, the monarchy for some long time now have shown their preference for homoeopathic medical care. On the other hand, homoeopathy is far more widely accepted on the Continent of Europe than in the UK. For example, there are few small towns in France which do not have a homoeopathic pharmacy, and in the big cities they are seen in almost every main thoroughfare.

Further proof by negative acceptance of homoeopathy inasmuch as the lower potencies do contain actual material substance is afforded by the regulations emanating from the appropriate department of that collective European emporium of wisdom and sagacity and hopefully other positive human qualities – the EEC Commission in Brussels. Homoeopathic remedies are licensed for manufacture and supply within the Community in all potencies, but all those remedies made from substances classified as poisons, that is, if they are not on the General Sales List and may therefore not be bought over the counter in a pharmacy, cannot be prescribed or supplied to patients other than by registered medical personnel. All medicines below the 4 CH potency (30 in UK terms) come into this category. The inference is that no material substance is contained in potencies higher than 4 CH. These are therefore considered safe and non-toxic in material terms. What is contained in these high potencies is more or less quietly ignored, but energy it is and sometimes very powerful energy too. Dr Leon Vannier, an eminent French homoeopath, referred to Homoeopathy as 'Medicine Atomique'.

Prana, 'chi, vital-energy, orgone energy, the five cosmo-physical energies, the patterned energy of the potentized homoeopathic remedy – are they all one and same thing? Or is it, in the final analysis, the spiritual energy which equates with the Buddha mind or, within the Christian context, the Grace of God?

We will leave it at that – the question unanswered – for who can answer it but oneself, by one's own interpretation and level of understanding. The labels do not matter – this energy is timeless and all-pervading, manifesting and functioning at every conceivable level of the living process.

Homoeopathy can therefore be described as being a system of energy-medicine par excellence. It is holistic and its mode of action and application is concerned equally with psyche and soma and by addressing its influence to what might be called the Inner Form.

Homoeopathic Principles and the Five Elements

As in Tantra there is a homoeopathic principle inasmuch as 'passion is passion's remedy', i.e. on the basis of 'like cures like', Tibetan Medicine may in one sense be said to be homoeopathic. This is because fundamentally both the disorders treated on the level of the Five Elements (and therefore the five cosmo-physical energies) and the medication employed has the same composition. In practice however the law of dissimilarity also pertains as well as the law of similarity. (See Chapter 3, p. 38) Homoeopathic diagnosis places great emphasis on the 'Modalities' – that is, questioning the patient, sometimes very exhaustively, about reactions to environmental factors: heat, cold, damp, wind, thunder, various foods; and the interrogation resembles enormously the twenty-nine classic and additional questions put to patients by Tibetan physicians. The 'Modalities' are in effect the expression of the actions and inter-reactions of the Five Elements both within, in the case of the human psycho-physical organism, and without, regarding environmental influence. Moreover both homoeopathy and Tibetan medicine place great importance on what are called the 'Mental Symptoms' and also the 'Constitutions'.

Homoeopathic Correspondences to Tridosha and the Three Humours

Many years ago I came across a truly remarkable work by Dr Benoytosh Bhattacharya – *The Science of Tridosha, The Three Cosmic Elements in Homoeopathy*.[4] Born in 1896 in India, Dr Bhattacharya was a well qualified and extremely cultured physician. It was he who was the first to consistently apply with great success the Ayurvedic doctrine of Tridosha to homoeopathy.

In the preface to Dr Bhattacharya's book, Howard D. Stangle says: 'What then is Tridosha?'. What, then, *is* Tridosha? It is, we are informed, a Sanskrit word comprised of two particles, tri (three) and dosha (fault), literally, 'the three faults'. That is, Tridosha treats the three elements in the human body most likely to become deranged and produce disease. Tridosha is the science of these three elements. In a sense it might be said that the elements of Air, Fire and Water, which are the inner motors of the outer garment of the human body, are like the thought, will and feeling of the human intelligence. They are its three main factors in life. These three forces, called Vata, Pitta and Kapha, with their subdivisions, belong within the sum total of human energies. But the author has nowhere said that they are representative of all the human forces. Their full triple meaning has been expanded in the chapters devoted to their elucidation, namely, Chapters ii, iii and iv.

In the development of the terms Fire and Water throughout the book, it will be observed that polarity is indicated, the poles positive and negative of all forms of energy and matter; and air considered as representing the neutral or axial centre common to both. Standard homoeopathic practice uses these terms under different designations, referring to them as the Hot and Cold temperaments of persons and, also, in the still closer comparison of Grauvogl, as the Oxygenoid, Hydrogenoid, and Carbo, nitrogenous constitutions. These latter relate both to medicines and to man. But until now, the finer shades of differentiation into which such forces fall appear not to have been given their proper recognition.

It will be found that the Tridosha system also embraces Hering's doctrine of the law of direction of cure, which asserts that diseases disappear in the reverse order of their coming, and 'from within outwards and from above downwards'. Tridosha clarifies the idea of cure, it points to the principle or the why of the passage 'from within to without' of disease causes and unnatural vibrations which have so evident a share in man's life.

Man is a dynamic being. His diseases are dynamic forces. Disease in all cases is the consequence of some derangement, and derangement is a disturbance of normal polarities, called in Ayurveda 'fire and water'. Normal polarity of the cell and its invisible energizing properties in this sense means simply magnetic alignment or arrangement of all the component particles of the cell. Disease, physically considered, can be nothing more than an upsetting of the normal condition, which is magnetic derangement of particles. A restoring of forces to normal is equal to a restoring of all constituent parts to a correct state of function. This is equilibrium, or health. Derangement, as the author shows, is first to be looked for among the fifteen finer forces, within the electro-vital fluids and functions of the human nature. These forces are being investigated today by means of techniques in use in the science of electronics.

It will be noted that the Three Faults correspond with the Three Humours, and are identical with the Three Humours of Tibetan medicine:

```
  rLung   –  Air      =  Vat
               (Wind)
mKhris-pa  –  Bile     =  Pit
  Bad-kan  –  Phlegm   =  Kaf
```

Remember (Chapter 3) that the Three Humours relate to the Five Elements as follows:

```
Air    =  Wind, which gives movement and dynamism
Fire   =  Bile, provides energy and heat
Earth  =  gives Extension (Expansion)
          through growth                            ⎫
Water  =  gives Cohesion (Contraction)    ⎬ together = Phlegm
          necessary to form                         ⎭
```
The fifth Element Space = is all pervading and represents the starting point of all phenomena and constructions which subsequently disintegrate and dissolve back into Space.

The fifteen 'finer forces' referred to are identical to the fifteen humours (five Winds, five Biles and five Phlegms). The rest is a matter of balance and order, exactly in the same way as it is described in Tibetan medicine. As Howard D. Stangle says:

> the chief point enunciated is, if balance is maintained in the body among its fifteen forces, or its three elements, there will be no disease. The upsetting of this balance may constitute either an excess or a deficiency of a particular element or elements. But if all the forces can be strengthened or balanced, there is no possibility of disease lingering in the system. But the

Table 8 Some important correlations and correspondences between homoeopathy, Tridosha and the Three Humours

Systems of medicine		Wind (Air)	Bile	Phlegm
	Tibetan medicine	Wind (Air)	Bile	Phlegm
	Ayurveda (Hindu medicine)	Air (Vat)	Fire (Pit)	Water (Kaf)
	Unani (Greco-Arabic medicine)	Hawa	Khun (Blood & Fire)	Balgum (Phlegm/Water)
Mental correspondences		thought – vital powers	will	feeling
Behaviour		fast	average	slow
Time of day		afternoon	noon	morning
Seasons		rains	autumn	spring
Hindu Deities & colours		Vishnu (blue)	Brahma (red)	Mahavesvara (white)
Electro-magnetic		neutron	electron	proton

diseaseless condition of the outer body is consistently dependent on the harmonious functioning taking place in the dynamic field itself, that is within the Inner Form.

Medicines likewise are possessed of their dynamic counterparts. The homoeopathic medicines which contain all the three elements of Vat (Air), Pit (Fire) and Kaf (Water) have the faculty of strengthening all the elements of the dynamic field of the body, and are able to aid all the fifteen genii (forces) in their maintenance of health. This applies equally to foods. To sum up, the terms Fire and Water as used in Tridosha correspond to the Hot and Cold diseases or disorders of Tibetan medicine and the Hot and Cold temperaments of classical homoeopathy. Some important correlations and correspondences between homoeopathy, Tridosha and the Three Humours are stated in Table 8.

Diseases are classified similarly in Tridosha as in Tibetan medicine, which is understandable since 'Tridosha *IS* the basis of Tibetan medicine, just as it is (with different implications) in Ayurveda' (Barry Clark).[5]

The classification of medicines and foods according to their element and fifteen-force content has been meticulously carried out and classified by Dr Bhattacharya. The 'modalities' and 'temperaments' of classical homoeopathy are used to decide and designate these properties. Dr Bhattacharya gives examples:

> Homoeopathic medicines having an aggravation between the hours of 2 and 6 by day and night are all air medicines.
> Pulsatilla has an aggravation in the afternoon, and therefore it is an air medicine. Thuja and Apis mel. are aggravated between the hours of 3 and 6 in the afternoon, and therefore they are air medicines.

The Six Jewels

Mention must be made of the 'Six Jewels of Homoeopathic Remedies' (Bhattacharya), which contain all three cosmo-physical energies and the fifteen forces. They are in fact eight which are classified as six accordingly:

1. Ammonium Carbonicum
   Ammonium Muriaticum
2. Baptisia
3. Camphora
4. Crocus Sativa
5. Ferrum Metallicum
   Ferrum Phosporicum
6. Sepia

As with all homoeopathic remedies they can be prescribed either by:

(a) classical repertorizing in the time-honoured way, probably the only acceptable method to the classical homoeopath

(b) repertorizing by computer (special computers exist for the purpose)
(c) pulse-diagnosis and questioning
(d) divination, by radiesthesia, radionics, etc.

Similarly foods which contain all the three 'elements' with the fifteen principles embedded in them. (Bhattacharya)

These are:
1. Cream
2. Milk (fresh)
3. Fish (fresh)
4. Black pepper

These have the power to strengthen all the fifteen principles in the body and keep them in a sound and healthy condition. But in their use the Middle Path is to be followed.

It is hardly necessary to add that milk, cream and fish are the best life-giving foods which nature has provided for mankind as a whole. Those who practise Yoga (meditation) subsist on milk alone, since it has all the properties to nourish the whole body. The manner in which cows are being destroyed threatens this precious food almost with extinction. The monks of India who lead a terribly irregular and unhygienic life, are habituated to take seven seeds of black pepper early in the morning and drink a little water after it. This is their tonic, this is their medicine, and strange as it may seem, these monks keep remarkably fit. The black pepper has the power to strengthen all the fifteen principles in the human body and keep them in a healthy condition. The secret of black pepper was well known to the monks. What the monks could do, all others also can do.

In view of the peculiar material difficulties in procuring and maintaining supplies of Tibetan medicines, aspiring practitioners in the West of that system, and especially if they be homoeopaths, can use the homoeopathic Materia Medica according to Tridosha, instead. There is no problem, homoeopathic remedies are freely available everywhere.

Electro-Homoeopathie

An interesting and relevant model of homoeopathic medicine is to be found in the *Vade-Mecum de l'Electro-Homoeopathie* by Count César Mattei, Bologna, Italy. My own copy is in the French language and unfortunately bears no date. The format and obvious age of the paper indicate that the edition is most probably late nineteenth century.

Count Mattei describes Five Constitutions:

1. Angiotic
2. Sanguin
3. Lymphatic
4. Tuberculinic
5. Cancerinic

Also Three Temperaments:

1. Nervous — which corresponds with rLung — Air or Wind
2. Sanguin } — which corresponds with mKhris-pa — Angiotic } Bile
3. Lymphatic } — which corresponds with Bad-kan — Tuberculinic } Phlegm

The author also describes Five Energies that manifest through the body as 'Électricités-végétales'. The adjective 'vegetative' would seem perhaps to translate better, thus conveying rather the sense that is most probably meant, i.e. 'basic biological-function energies'.

The Five Electricities correspond with five colours as follows:

Red Electricity } are positive in polarity
Blue Electricity }
Green Electricity } are negative in polarity
Yellow Electricity }
White Electricity is Neutral

This gives a group of three:

red/blue – positive
green/yellow – negative
white – neutral

Pharmacological action

For Stimulating – Red Electricity is indicated for the Lymphatic and Tuberculinic Constitutions and Temperaments (Phlegm).

For Relaxing – Yellow Electricity is indicated for the Nervous Constitutions and Temperaments (Wind).

For Contracting – Blue Electricity is indicated for the Sanguin Constitutions and Temperaments (Bile).

As an Antiseptic – Green Electricity is indicated for the Cancerinic constitutions.

As a Supportive – White Electricity is indicated for all constitutions and temperaments and especially where there is great weakness and other Electricities are ineffective.

(On pages 37–8 of his book Count Mattei gives the correspondence of his various remedies with the Electricities.)

Remedies are applied in the usual homoeopathic way in the form of:

1. Globules internally, and externally
2. Ointments, lotions, injections, bathing, compresses and gargles.

Altogether another interesting combination of *threes* and *fives*, numbers of great significance, which together with *seven*, *eight*, *ten*, *twelve*, *twenty-one* and *one hundred and eight* are found in Buddha Dharma and other religions and philosophies, particularly those of oriental origin, sometimes referred to as 'esoteric'.

14

Osteopathy I

Osteopathy: the Perfect Complement to Tibetan Medicine

Osteopathy has been given more prominence, as far as the relevant similarities both in theory and clinical practice are concerned, over the other forms of medicine and particularly occidental. This is simply because, being primarily an osteopath, I am more qualified to talk about osteopathy than the other disciplines. Long experience of both practising osteopathy and, to a lesser degree, the Buddha Dharma in the Tibetan tradition, has resulted in three chapters instead of the one that was originally planned.

The blanket term 'manual medicine' in the West includes a number of disciplines and techniques which are concerned with the manipulation of body tissues with therapeutic intent. Classically osteopathic treatment is in the first instance primarily directed to the musculo-skeletal system itself: bones, joints, articulations, ligaments, muscles, etc., usually considering them as an ensemble. Sometimes however particular emphasis is given in treatment of the whole to one or other of these aspects – ligamentous, muscular, for example, as the case may be. Occasionally they may be treated in isolation, but this is exceptional.

Other forms of 'manual medicine' (chiropractic excepted) tend to fall into either a medical auxiliary or adjuvant context or may be practised by 'therapists'. Classical and other forms of massage, reflex-techniques, acupressure, and shiatsu are examples of these.

Osteopathy on the other hand is a system of medicine in its own right. The formal training involved includes the full range of medical diagnostics as well as the osteopathic diagnostic procedures themselves. Such practitioners are therefore not only trained to manipulate both skilfully and safely in the traditional sense, but are also able to make their own independent diagnostic assessment of their patients. Osteopaths, however, while regarding the spine as the central-point of their attention, also give equal prominence to the role of the extremities and peripheral joints and articulations, within the total holistic mechanical and functional arrangement of the musculo-skeletal system.

As will be seen later, diagnosis and treatment extend today into bioenergetic concepts and procedures, which again differentiate it from the other forms of manual medicine. Moreover, osteopathy addresses itself to the functional element in disease, and while it postulates a mechanical theory of disease it is not mechanistic as such, either in its philosophy, principles or practice, nor is it totally vitalist. Disturbed body mechanics can give rise to functional disturbances and vice versa, as will be seen later.

Historical Aspects

Osteopathy is a system of manual medicine which originated in the USA in the 1870s. The founder, Dr Andrew Taylor Still, born in 1830, was the son of a clergyman who also practised medicine.

The first osteopathic school was opened by Still in Kirksville, Missouri. Osteopathy was brought to the UK by graduates of this school around 1902/3. Dr J. Martin Littlejohn, who had been first Professor of Physiology and second Dean at the Kirksville School, returned to Britain where he later founded the present British School of Osteopathy in 1918. The European School of Osteopathy, Maidstone, Kent (England) was originally opened in Paris in 1951 as the French School of Osteopathy, which came to the UK in 1965. Both the BSO and the ESO, together with the London College of Osteopathic Medicine, are the three major training establishments in the UK. The Université Paris-Nord (Faculty of Medicine) recognizes the ESO inasmuch as their osteopathic faculty is drawn from that of the ESO.

It was probably as a result of Still's intuition as a child, that he eventually conceived the idea of osteopathy.[1] When he was very young he used to suffer from violent headaches. At the age of ten, while playing one day in the garden, he developed one of these headaches and laid down to rest close to his swing. Feeling that he would be more comfortable if his head was supported, he rested it on the rope of the swing in such a way that it was supported just below the base of the skull. After a few moments to his astonishment, his headache disappeared. He probably gave it no more thought at the time, except to resort to this practice whenever a headache came on.

Later Andrew Still studied medicine and graduated from the College of Medicine and Surgery in Kansas City. Although he was trained as an allopathic physician he nevertheless had a consuming passion to study the human structure. His first opportunity to do so came when he was able to examine Red Indian skeletons. A little later, during the Civil War, he served as an army medical orderly. This experience gave him plenty of opportunity to examine human structure and particularly the spinal column. He began to notice a connection between the usual illnesses and certain structural anomalies. It then dawned on him why, as a child, he was able to cure his headaches by supporting his neck on the swing. The weight of his head on the rope had caused the tense neck muscles to relax by a process of inhibition, which in turn had decongested the circulation of his head and the headaches had disappeared – such was his reasoning.

Still's Principles (or Precepts)

This discovery led Still in 1872 to formulate several principles which to this day still constitute the basis of the practice of contemporary osteopathic medicine. The first Principle states that 'Structure Governs Function', principally if the former is disturbed through its potential physio-pathologic influence on the circulation of body fluids. This may be both mechanical and/or reflex, involving changes of vasomotor tone expressed through autonomic nervous system imbalance ranging from relative hyperaemia to ischaemia. All tissues, both musculo-skeletal and visceral (i.e.

wherever there is a vasomotor influence) can be potentially involved. Hence the second Principle – 'The Rule of the Artery is Supreme', which was Still's way in those days of expressing the paramount importance of circulatory disturbances in ill health and pathology. The third Principle – 'Find it, fix it and leave it alone' – is an admonition for minimal treatment, i.e. that amount of treatment which is necessary and no more. 'It' refers to the somatic dysfunction (osteopthic-lesion). Still laid down a further principle – 'the body makes its own medicines', i.e. providing that all homeostatic mechanisms are functioning normally and adequate nutrition is operative.

More recently certain 'trigger-sites' in the vertebral column have been shown to be associated with the neuro-endocrine system, namely the segments CI, II and III, DIV/V, DIX, LV/SACRUM. The first Principle is also found to operate in reverse – i.e. that function (and particularly dysfunction) can influence and sometimes actually cause structural change. For example – hypertrophy both musculo-skeletal and visceral can occur as the result of constant hyperfunction. Changes of posture, functional at first, but eventually resulting in simple musculo-skeletal pathology – fibrosis or arthrosis – may be caused by a prolonged and continuous emotional reaction to stress, e.g. the rigid, withdrawn morphology of chronic anxiety.

Still's researches led him to discover what is known today as the 'somatic dysfunction' (formerly described as the 'osteopathic lesion'), which could be systematically palpated. He evolved the various manual procedures, both diagnostic and therapeutic, which laid the basis for present-day osteopathic diagnosis and technique.

The Somatic-Dysfunction (Osteopathic Lesion)

In its broadest sense a 'somatic dysfunction' is: a disturbance of the musculo-skeletal system that may express dysfunction on any level and may even be a factor in the development of organic disease.

Osteopathy regards the human's change from a quadruped to a biped stance as one of the main predisposing aetiological factors in human ailments. Add to this the effect of macro- and microtraumata, either acute or chronic, and mechanical imbalance quickly follows. In the biped stance, gravity has a continuously deleterious effect on man's structure. For instance:

(1) The intervertebral discs and the apophyseal joints of the spine have become weight-bearing, tending to make the junction areas extremely unstable, especially the lumbo-sacral and sacro-iliac articulations.

(2) It is on account of the continuous strain at the level of these articulations that low-back pain and sciatica are so common. This constitutes a typical osteopathic mechanical lesion of the low back, and is very amenable to osteopathic treatment. Furthermore, gravity tends to make the abdominal and pelvic viscera, including the diaphragm, sag inferiorly. This predisposes to visceroptosis, hernia, portal hypertension, haemorrhoids, constipation, varix and other conditions due to intra-abdominal compression and stasis.

Much of the cardio-vascular system is obliged to function against gravity, and equally has to constantly adapt to changing posture. Similarly with the respiratory system, the bronchi must drain against gravity, i.e. by means of coughing, sneezing and the actions of the ciliated epithelium.

(3) Should there be any excessive or mechanical distortion on a spinal articulation, the weight of gravity will tend to hold the joint in stress, usually at an extreme point of its normal range of movement, and reduced mobility ensues.

This becomes one type of 'somatic-dysfunction' – the structural-mechanical. This term also includes any state of stress involving any structure and its function. For example, articulations other than in the spine may be included, such as in the extremities; other examples include the fascial planes, muscles, legs, viscera, endocrine glands, etc. Briefly, this type of somatic-dysfunction may be described as a modification of normal joint movement which is of vital importance in the spinal column. This is not meant to imply that change in the apposition of the joint surfaces is sufficient to describe the somatic-dysfunction. All struc-tures surrounding and attached to the vertebral area are involved and such terms as stress, strain, thickening, shortening, swelling, etc., give the clue to what is really a physio-pathological and mechanical condition and not a mere anatomical deviation, although, of course, these can and do occur, and it is from these several factors, collectively or singly, that the functional activity of the body begins to suffer. Provided the analogy is kept in perspective, the spinal areas may be regarded as a series of 'junction boxes' which play a leading part in the regulation and control of the great nervous and circulatory systems of the body, and it is here that disturbance may originate or where primary organic disorder may lead to break-down in the co-ordination of the spinal control.[2]

Somatic-dysfunctions of recent occurrence are usually designated as being 'acute'; long-standing somatic-dysfunctions are described as 'chronic'. Both types can occur in the same patient, the chronic developing from the acute, or the acute can manifest, from time to time, within the chronic state. The point to be made clear is that the somatic-dysfunction state is progressive and that the acute condition is often an expression of compensatory failure. Whatever type it is that we have to consider, the potential causes are several and must be traced to their source. Primary somatic-dysfunctions frequently arise from accidents, blows, torsional stress, improper posture, nutritional errors, infection, or from metabolic retention and auto-toxaemia. Mental and emotional factors such as anxiety, fear, frustration, resentment, etc., may also lead to disturbance of the spinal balance. Whatever the etiological factor responsible for the state of disease, whether it be traumatic, postural, dietetic or psychological, the functioning of the body is impaired, and if this is continued over long periods, organic tissue changes are likely to occur. From the osteopathic point of view, the osteopathic somatic-dysfunction represents the sole etiological factor in this vicious circle of functional and organic disorder, and it is here that corrective and normalizing influences of manipulation can be bought to bear, to restore the natural defences and to allow the self-regulating tendency of the body to come into operation. Therein lies the rationale of Still's original hypotheses. The role of the osteopath is to normalize

Table 9 Classification of somantic-dysfunctions

Etiology	Designation of Somatic-Dysfunction	
TRAUMA – either macro, micro- or in combination	Somatico-somatic lesion Somatico-visceral lesion Somatico-psychic lesion	directly arising from *without*
visceral pathology, infections, emotional stresses and strains, and particularly conflict	Viscero-somatic Psycho-somatic	directly arising from *within*

structural and functional disturbances by manual treatment plus such other adjuvant procedures as may be necessary in the given case.

Table 9 represents the full classification of somatic-dysfunctions in relation to their etiology, as understood and taught at the European School of Osteopathy.

The Facilitated Segment

All that has been said in this respect may be additionally expressed in terms particularly original to Denslow and Korr[3] concerning the 'facilitated segment'. By definition an inter-vertebral somatic-dysfunction means that there is a tissue stretch on one side and a shortening on the other. All the para-vertebral structures (including muscles, ligaments, etc.) are richly supplied with sensory nerve endings, which are sensitive to such changes of tension and are of the non-adapting type.

For example, let us suppose that as a result of trauma or physical irritation a vertebra side bent on the one below. The proprioceptors on the lengthened side (neuro-muscular spindle, golgi tendon receptors) will continuously bombard the spinal cord segment to which they are related. We are here assuming that the upper vertebra has become immobilized on the one below in side bending, this being called in osteopathy a 'spinal side-bending rotation dysfunction' (rotation is usually complementary to side-bending).

Denslow, Korr and others have shown experimentally that this afferent bombardment facilitates the neuronal pool of the related spinal cord segment. This facilitation implies that these neurones are maintained at or near threshold level. In the neuronal pool, there are three important types of neurones: motor, sensory and autonomic. Korr described how facilitation through the different fibres affects all three types and I shall discuss them in turn.

Denslow has shown that this leads to a hypertonicity and hyper-irritability of the muscles supplied by that segment. This will lead to biochemical changes within the muscle structures. A patient so affected would present with constant muscle tension which might be misunderstood as resulting from emotional stress, which it could be of course, whereas in this case it is not – the cause is mechanical and physical.

Pain threshold is lowered in the muscles, skin, periosteum, ligament and fascia supplied from that segment. Hyperaesthesia is experienced, and where the etiology is traumatic the patient will continue to feel pain for an unusually long time after the effects of the trauma have ceased to operate.

Sudomotor activity is increased in the segmentally related dermatome, this being an important cutaneous sign of a vertebral somatic-dysfunction. The resultant sympatheticotonia leads to vaso-constriction in the segmentally related dermatome and viscera. It is this sympatheticotonia which is thought to be the most deleterious consequences of this facilitation. The sympathetic neurons of that segment become indefinitely susceptible to the least stimulus, psychological or physical, being constantly at or near threshold levels.

Normally the sympathetics have only an intermittent effect on the viscera, as during stress and exercise. However, under these circumstances the sympathetics stimulate the viscera, not only during stress and exercise, but also they are facilitated, in response to any increased nervous activity in the body.

If we take for example the gastro-intestinal tract, this sympathetic facilitation results in decreased peristalsis and glandulo-motor activity as well as vaso-constriction in the gastro-intestinal tract. Osteopathy regards this is an important aetiological factor in much physio-pathology involving the GIT some of which is often allergy related in the susceptible individual.

The Traditional Emphasis on the Role of the Circulatory System

Osteopathy primarily stresses the role of the circulatory system in health and disease and is traditionally concerned with the Outer Form of the human phenomenon, i.e. the structuro-mechanical aspects of the physical body, in terms of the elements of the musculo-skeletal system already mentioned, plus the fascia and connective-tissues which bind and hold together the various organs, glands, vessels (arteries, veins and lymphatics). Here the physical nervous system, which has two aspects – central and autonomic, together with the endocrines correlates and harmonizes physical homeostasis in terms of structure governing function. All these aspects are subject to the physical laws of mechanics, hydraulics, thermo-dynamics, electro-magnetism and electronics, in terms of the western sciences of anatomy, physiology, biochemistry, etc. Traditionally the manual techniques of diagnosis and treatment are primarily mechanical. As will be seen later this structural-mechanical approach, which is in effect a second phase in the evolution and development of osteopathy, belongs basically to the first fifty years of this century.

However, more recently in osteopathy there has been a shift or more correctly perhaps a marked swing virtually to the polar opposite, i.e. away from the traditionally structural-mechanical basis to the functional, bioenergetic concepts of practice, with the development of new techniques which would appear on the face of it to bear little or no resemblance to the traditional mechanically-based manipulative procedures.

Sutherland's Discovery of the Cranial Rhythmic Impulse

The critical turning-point in this otherwise heavily grounded structural-mechanical manual medicine came with the revolutionary and indeed riveting discovery some fifty odd years ago by an American osteopathic physician W.G. Sutherland of the Cranial Rhythmic Impulse (CRI)[4] although this did not have any great impact on the profession until the 1950s. This is an intrinsic, rhythmic pulsation involving an expansion-contraction, flexion-extension phenomenon occurring at approximately 10–14 cycles per minute (some authorities say 8–12). While it is primarily designated as being cranial in its basic manifestation, it nevertheless involves the whole body. With little training and average sensitivity it may be felt by anyone. The subtle changes, however, and modifications relating to a diverse number of altered functions and tissue-states in the body, and equally subtle variations in mento-emotional tonus in totally holistic relationship, is quite a different matter and requires a long and patient training and practice. The mastery of osteopathic diagnosis through the CRI is certainly most demanding, as is pulse-taking in the Tibetan, Chinese and Ayurvedic systems of medicine.

To further elucidate, the inherent, periodic rhythms of pulsations of the body, having a frequency on the order of 0.2 Hz., have been designated the cranial rhythmic impulse, whose amplitude and directions may vary. The cranial rhythmic impulse (CRI) has been described as being propagated through the body as a wave of minutely perceptible motion. Somatic-dysfunction in this conceptual model is expressed as perturbations in the rate, amplitude, direction or symmetry of these impulses. Axiomatic in this system is the assumption that in the healthy body, variations in the rate, amplitude, direction of CRI occur in regular, predictable cycles, and that there is an overall symmetry in the way in which CRI waves are transmitted. It is clear that this conceptualization is best described as a fluid mechanism through which waves may be transmitted.

In the fascial-tension model, the fascia includes the cranial and spinal dura and its reflections. Anatomic continuity provides a mechanical, geometric system that can be described in terms of its behaviour in response to the inherent motions (e.g. CRI) of the body in terms of its response to test motions imposed on the system by the examiner. Treatment in the context of this model may be done with direct positioning, utilizing the inherent forces of the body to effect correction of inappropriate tightness in the fascia. Some osteopaths conceptualize and utilize what to them is a visible or palpable field of energy around the body. Their understanding and interpretation of perturbations of this energy field are based on a theoretical model of bioenergy.

Harold I. Magoun Sr. DO, a primary researcher in the field of cranial osteopathy, mentioned that during brain surgery four pulsations of that organ have been observed. One co-ordinates with the cardiac rhythm, i.e. the pulse beats, another with the breathing or the respiration. Normally there is a co-ordination between these two which expresses itself in a ratio of $4\frac{1}{2}$–1. The origin of the other two pulsations is not known generally to physiologists. Sutherland's view is that the third and fourth pulsations are due to 'the innate motility of the central nervous system and the accompanying fluctuations of the cerebro-spinal fluid within its enclosed container'. Sutherland quotes Dr John A. MacDonald:

> All animate tissues are in constant rhythmic motion. The brain
> is not a quiet lifeless mass of nerve tissues. Its convolutions coil
> and uncoil and the ventricles dilate and contract in rhythmic
> unison with the alternating cranial-articular membranous
> activity in relation to respiration. Hence abnormal fixations
> occurring in the normal range of cranial articular membranous
> activity also limit brain and ventricle movement.[5]

This is important in view of the fact that all the physiological centres including that of respiration are located within the floor of the fourth ventricle of the brain.

The other two pulsations mentioned above are related to but at the same time independent of the cardiac/respiratory rhythms and pulsations. For instance if the breath is deliberately held, the CRI continues uninterruptedly. Similarly with other biorhythms, the variations and cycles of which may be measured or assessed by

Biorhythmic Calculators, which constitute a fifth category of intrinsic energy pulsation. To re-cap:

The 5 innate	1. Cardiac
intrinsic	2. Respiratory
Pulsations	3. CNS (Central Nervous System)
	4. CSF (Cerebro-Spinal Fluid)
	5. Biorhythms

As mentioned previously the CRI involves the whole body, with the cranio-sacral (head-pelvis) mechanism as the focus and it manifests this continuously throughout life in the form of a flexion-extension (expansion-contraction) movement which takes place in the spheno-basilar articulation. The body changes which are palpable to the trained osteopath are as follows:

In FLEXION	*In EXTENSION*
External rotation of the whole body.	Internal rotation of the whole body.
Head is shorter and broader, particularly the occiput.	Head is longer and narrower.
Extremities and feet and hands are in external rotation.	Extremities and feet and hands are in internal rotation.
All fascia is felt to be on tension.	All fascia slacken off.
Note: Corresponds mentally with extraversion and *action*, and inspiration (breathing).	*Note*: Corresponds mentally with introversion and *passivity*, and expiration (breathing).

The Four Evolutionary Stages of Osteopathy

There have been four evolutionary states of osteopathy:

1. The formative and primarily developmental stage from 1872 to approximately 1920+.
2. The great structural-mechanical period from 1920+ to 1960.

3. The cranial/functional phase from 1960 to 1975 approximately.
4. The middle-way, holistic model which gives, as Still did during the founding stage, equal emphasis to the dynamic structural-functional — functional-structural aspects in diagnosis and technique.

In the twentieth century, influenced by the great urge to explain everything scientifically, Still's successors continued to develop osteopathy in objective, mechanical, physio-biochemical terms. This second period, the great structural-mechanical age of osteopathy was responsibile for the development and consolidation of a very mechanical bias in osteopathic diagnosis and technique, heavily influenced in some quarters by orthopaedic thinking. The 'bone out of place in the spine' and 'clicking it back' became the overriding consideration and threatened at one point in the post-war period to virtually replace Still's original hypotheses and concepts.

The swing back to the mid-line, the fourth phase, is here. It started with the third period in the evolution and development of osteopathic medicine which begun with Sutherland's discovery of the Cranial Rhythmic Impulse. This in fact manifested as the polar opposite of the second mechanistic period and which at one point almost became a hyper-functional technique phase.

Contemporary interpretations of the same phenomena that preoccupied Still and his co-workers, plus Sutherland's discovery, have now given rise to concepts very similar to those of the first stage. These emphasize, as did Still at the beginning, the dynamic relationships relative to the functional and structural aspects of the body-mind complex and their role in health and disease.

Osteopathic Diagnosis

Osteopathic diagnosis as such involves a total structuro-mechanical-functional examination and consists of the following procedures:

(a) *Inspection* – static and dynamic, standing and sitting; seeing through the patients as well as observing their outer form.

(b) *Palpation* – involving all tissues: bone, joint-capsules, muscles and ligaments in terms of normal and abnormal anatomy and using visualization.

(c) *Mobility-Testing* – particularly the vertebral articulations, visualizing the normal and abnormal in terms of articular physiology.

(d) *'Listening'* – with the hands to: the CRI cranial rhythmic impulse, other body-rhythms, bio-energetic variations, changes of emotional tonus and X factors according to the intuition and sensitivity of the practitioner concerned.

In this way the osteopath seeks to identify both quantitatively and qualitatively the presence of somatic-dysfunctions relative to the particular clinical problem in the given patient.

It follows that this diagnostic assessment involves all levels – structural, physiological and bio-energetic. By 'putting the mind inside the body' as well as observing and ascertaining external departures from normal structure the osteopath is concerned, above all, with looking for the 'functional element' in whatever the departure from normal health may be in the particular patient. Osteopaths are also trained in general medicine, and a medical and/or surgical diagnosis is made wherever necessary with recourse to X-rays and 'Path. Lab.' procedures. This is additional to the osteopathic diagnosis as such.

Osteopathic Technique

Manual medicine techniques are ubiquitous and osteopathic technique is as unique as it is diverse. There are many conceptual technique models but each contains certain essential characteristics which reflect the essentially osteopathic thinking behind their rationale.

A new student in a class at the ESO, to whom I was recently lecturing, asked the question – 'What makes a procedure, either in diagnosis or technique, osteopathic as such?' My immediate answer was: because it evolved within and forms part of long usage in a traditional osteopathic context — an immediate classroom response! Not incorrect of course but incomplete. As noted above, it is the osteopathic thinking, superficially conceptual of course, that determines the particular label 'osteopathic'. On a deeper contemplative level Still's precepts lead one to appreciate the strong underlying element of the pure intuitive knowledge (prajna — yeshes) involved in osteopathic thinking. This applied not only to Still, the founder, but to all the other great pioneers of osteopathy, as will be seen later. Osteopathic technique has therefore evolved on a continuously changing basis since Still first conceived and invented so to speak, the original manual procedures known subsequently as osteopathic technique.

The four developmental stages mentioned earlier, arbitrarily delineate this continuously evolving process. In terms of osteopathic technique they are as follows:

Stage 1

Historically evidence shows that Still's original technique was as functional in its approach and application as it was structural.

Stage 2

The pendulum swung well over to the structural-mechanical concept and usage, based on the solid, comfortable and reassuring foundations of anatomy, physiology, biochemistry, etc. GOT (General Osteopathic Technique) and other variants of what we now call structural-mechanical technique came to their own during this period.

Stage 3

This represents the swing in the totally opposite direction, not necessarily involving a rejection of the thinking pertinent to Stage 2, but certainly giving rise to the feeling of great adventure involving an exciting journey into the unknown — the world of metaphysics and the exploration of the noumenal as opposed to the relatively dull and routine of the phenomenal. Cranial and Functional Techniques are particularly identified with this evolutionary stage of osteopathy.

Stage 4

This is sometimes alluded to as 'the return to the source' (the osteopathic 'middle-way', back to the original structural-functional – functional-structural technique model of the founder Dr A.T. Still), the wheel of osteopathy having turned full cycle. There is one reservation of course, allowing for all that has been accumulated in osteopathic theory and practice since Still founded osteopathy in 1872: perhaps it is more correct to say that, in turning full cycle, osteopathy has also gone up one level on the evolutionary spiral.

General Osteopathic Treatment (GOT)

In ESO thinking this forms the solid basis, the earth-element in osteopathy. The structural-mechanical approach thus forms the solid basis of the first two years of training. The intuitive level is however by no means neglected; as mentioned in the section on diagnosis students are taught 'to put their minds into the tissues' and visualize the living anatomy and physiology together with the palpable functional energetic changes, i.e. appreciating the Wind (Air) element level particularly as it manifests in the solid matrix of the earth element, inasmuch as simple functional technique is also introduced modestly in the first two years. GOT seeks to evoke a circulatory response primarily at the level of the vaso-motor system and consists of moving tissues both hard and soft* through various movements relative to the anatomy and physiology, with the object of normalizing both function and tissue tone. In addition it acts as a stimulus to the re-attainment of a normal state, both concerning the musculo-skeletal tissues

---

* hard tissues – bones, tendons. When they degenerate there is a diminution of the Earth element and an increase in others, particularly the Water and Air elements. soft-tissues – muscles, ligaments, joint capsules, cartilages. When they degenerate there is an increase in the Earth element content and they become harder.

which are themselves being actually treated, as well as exerting a distant and reflex effect elsewhere within the totality. Relatively slow, repetitive movement using long-levers (e.g. legs and arms) is known as articulatory treatment. More speedy, sometimes 'high velocity' manoeuvres involving short-levers or even direct contact in this case on the spinal-bone (vertebra) being treated are known as adjustments or corrections. Traditionally the model of GOT judiciously combines both soft-tissue, articulatory and bony adjustments (or corrections) into one whole procedure. The therapeutic intent of the GOT operator is to structurally and mechanically re-balance weight-bearing and body mechanics and thus functionally restore the dynamic equilibrium of the whole person on all levels. These changes are primarily induced by the nature of the procedures which are imposed directly by the GOT practitioner until what is considered to be the 'norm' for that person is restored. This represents a kind of direct remodelling of nature's aberrations, in response to environmental changes and stimuli, and as such is primarily reductive as an approach. Nevertheless, it is holistic inasmuch that the part (or parts) are treated through the 'whole'.

Specific Adjusting Technique

Known but very little outside of the ESO, SAT is a minimal treatment model, non-reductive inasmuch as it relies totally on invoking a specific response throughout the whole homeostatic chain. This occurs particularly on the level of the proprioceptor system, involving either the more superficial neuro-circulatory mechanisms or the deeper neuro-hormonal level. The SAT practitioner does not impose a therapeutic solution. Rather, obstructions in the form of somatic-dysfunctions or 'osteopathic lesions' are systematically and progressively removed, thus invoking a direct homeostatic, and indeed a more than often spontaneous, response. SAT can be applied equally in a mechanical-structural or a functional way, throughout the whole spectrum of clinical requirement and is therefore universal in its approach. Self-regulating anabolic mechanisms and processes come into play, and structure and function re-balances on all levels. Sometimes this is a dramatic event, other times there is a more slow and progressive return to normal, which is usually punctuated by a series of aggravation or amelioration (in a homoeopathic sense) phases.

Functional Technique

Functional Technique (Indirect Positioning Technique) emerged in the osteopathic profession in the early 1950s, associated with Harold V. Hoover. It was taken up by the New England Academy of Applied Osteopathy, in particular by the Educational Committee under the Chairmanship of Charles H. Bowles. They held a series of study sessions over a number of years, reporting their work in the American Academy of Osteopathy Yearbook. One of the pioneers of this early work was Dr William L. Johnston, now Professor in the Department of Biomechanics, Michigan State University, College of Osteopathic Medicine.

Functional Technique essentially consists of guiding the patient through a series of controlled active movements, palpating at the suspected segment continuously to establish directions of progressive ease and progressive bind. The segment is then led through a pattern of motion to reduce the resistance to motion and thus, improve the segmental function.

Cranial Technique

Cranial Technique which logically emerged as the result of Sutherland's historic discovery, the inevitable swing to the opposite pole, has in the intervening years evolved considerably. Different interpretations of the phenomenon are based on the emphasis given to the various aspects of the anatomo-physiological-energetic whole person. Some workers interpret their diagnostic findings in terms of variations in membranous tonus. Others base their conclusions rather on body-fluid or bioenergetic considerations. Functional and fascial-unwinding techniques are associated but later developments.

To re-cap, there are at least three distinct conceptual models by which cranial manipulation may be applied:

1) The fluid model.
2) The fascial-tension model.
3) The bioenergy model.

Each contains its own definition of somatic-dysfunction.

Miscellaneous Osteopathic Techniques

Other osteopathic techniques taught at the ESO are Fascial-Unwinding, Muscle-Energy Technique (Mitchell) and Counter Strain Technique (Jones). Space does not allow description of these.

The suitability, either total or partial, of any or either of these techniques is dependent on many factors – the clinical problem, the biotypology of the particular patient in question, the temperament, personality and personal orientation and manual dexterity and handling ability of the osteopath in question. In the ESO all students are required to become competent and effective in Mechanical-Structural Technique first, before going on to the cranial and functional approaches. Since this involves moderation through the external examination system this avoids the criticism that Cranial Technique is a 'cop-out' for those who are unable to master the more traditional mechanical-structural techniques.

In the absence of any important mental/emotional block or particular pathology all osteopathic techniques, if competently applied in accordance with a valid osteopathic diagnosis as well as a medical one, are effective in suitable cases.

Still's Spiritual and Intuitive Insight into Healing

Andrew Taylor Still discovered what he called the principles of osteopathy, and laid down the fundamental precepts and founded osteopathy as an independent system of medicine in the mid-1980s. A devout Christian and a very spiritual man, he saw the perfection of the human body as a divine manifestation, fashioned by – to use his own words – The Great Architect of the Universe. His approach to patients and the treatment of the outer gross form reflected enormously, in a spiritual and metaphysical sense, the very evangelical Christian concepts of his time. In Chapter 15 his probably totally unconscious identification with the Tantric understanding of the Clear Light of the Void is discussed in some detail. Dr Still mystically referred to 'the highest known element in the human body' – something invisible yet it has the inherent quality of brilliant Light – Liquid Light[6] he called it. What other than the Clear Light of Shunyata? This spiritual and intuitive insight was not common solely to Still, nor was it confined only to his time. Many osteopathic pioneers over the years have been strongly endowed with it. Today osteopathy, in my belief, has taken on an even extra dimension, i.e. in terms of philosophy, additional to the primarily Western evangelical Christian environment in which it was born.

15

Osteopathy II

The Great Breath

Life begins with the act of Inspiration associated cosmically with the 'Great Breath'[1] – all pulsations are activated. There are differing religious, spiritual and philosophical interpretations of this phenomenon. Life also terminates with the involuntary act of Expiration and all pulsations stop. Preparatory to both states, embryology describes the beginning – be it either in a Western or Tibetan Buddhist tradition – and likewise the end, as in the *Tibetan Book of the Dead*.[2]

Macrocosmically, it is said that the Universe itself pulsates similarly. Indeed may not total human existence and function be merely expressing this microcosmically through its five fundamental pulsations,* i.e. noumenally rather than phenomenally? Perhaps this could also explain the nature of the dynamic qualities and behaviour of the three cosmic energies (humours), and similarly related energy variations in the radial pulses? Osteopaths are trained, as Sutherland says – 'to feel, think and see with their fingers' beyond and in between normal physiology and pathology, and not to just mechanically inspect and palpate the grosser and more static tissue states and their retrograde changes. May they not also be doing virtually the same thing as the Tibetan doctor, particularly in terms of pulse diagnosis?

---

* five fundamental pulsations – five cosmo-physical energies (Five Elements)

The Clinical Significance of Past Lives

Professor John Upledger, DO, formerly in charge of research in the Department of Biomechanics, Michigan State University claims that by means of Fascial-Unwinding Technique, it is possible to regress clinical subjects back into previous lifetimes and find operative causes (karmic) for illnesses in this present lifetime. Similar experiences have been carried out clinically by Denis Kelsey, MD, and his wife Joan Grant, authoress of *Many Lifetimes* and other books on reincarnation. The contributions in the linear multi-dimensional, rather than the purely horizontal and/or vertical links between etiology and disease manifestation by Edgar Cayce and Arther Guirdham, are also fundamental to these aspects of the total osteopathic medicine spectrum.

Structure/Function and the Significance of Tantra

Structure/Function

As inevitable as the swing of the polar opposites is the constant dynamism of everything in life always coming back to the mid-line, an expression very common in osteopathic jargon which expresses itself as a continuity of oscillation around its 'centre' or fixed-point. (See the 'Systems Theory' of Fritjof Capra,[3] and Chapter 3, p. 46, Lama Govinda.)

Beginning with Sutherland, osteopathy is no exception to this law of polarization. This age of contemporary osteopathic discovery marks a new era of radical departure from the old structural-mechanical concepts.

In terms of the newer knowledge and understanding, the first precept – 'Structure governs function' – is interpreted equally as 'function governs structure'. Dr Viola Frymann, an eminent American osteopathic physician, has pointed out that in reality 'structure is solidified motion (function)', to which may be added 'function (motion) is de-solidified structure'. Structure and function are therefore indivisible and are simply two aspects of the one expressed bioenergy, which in a Tantric sense is the expression of the inherent motility and particular qualities or 'be-ness' of all material forms, beings and things.

Psychic Channels or Pathways

In discussing the psychic channels or pathways (rtsa) in the human body, Guenther[4] explains this as follows:

> In the course of this analysis of the pathways we have had occasion to refer to another important feature in the picture of man's being, that is, motility (rlun,* vayu), which is defined as 'that which makes everything move'. It serves as the vehicle of the creative potentiality along the pathways. The basic meaning of the word rlun (vayu) is 'wind', and as breath, perceptible only at low temperatures, this easily suggests its use as a symbol of that which mediates between the invisible and the visible.
>
> However, breathing is only one form of motility which we can observe or sense throughout the working of our body. Here too, it would not be difficult to identify the various forms of motility described in the texts with what we call the circulatory, respiratory, digestive, eliminative, reproductive, endocrine, nervous and muscular systems. The texts themselves assert that between this picture of man's being and that of medicine there is a certain similarity. But this is not so much a problem of anatomy as of function, and in this connection it is interesting to note that the conative aspect of mind is stressed. Tantrism thus anticipates a trend in modern psychology.
>
> In the same way as the pathways pointed to motility, the latter refers beyond itself to creative potentiality to which reference has already been made by one of the names of the upper end of the central pathway, 'Pure Consciousness'. It is essential to note that yid (manas) always denotes mind before it has crystallized into consciousness in the sense in which we understand this latter term.
>
> In relation to creative potentiality, motility is seen from two angles, awareness-motility which serves as the vehicle of the three reaction potentialities,** and action-motility which is the carrier of the eighty reaction patterns. The distinction between

---

* 'rlun' is the same as 'rlung' because it should be spelt 'rlun' = Wind.

** The Three Humours

the pathways' motility and creative potentiality is, of course, not so strict as language seems to suggest. Actually all the three terms refer to one and the same process viewed from various angles. So also, what the text calls the 'common feature of psycho-organism and spirituality', and defines as the subtle identity and the reaction potentialities, out of which in course of evolution conscious experience develops, is the unique character of sentient life which in its awareness moves along certain ways. The Tantric texts again seem to have anticipated what Judson C. Herrick says on the basis of psycho-biology: 'Overt behaviour is movement of some sort. Movement is primordial and mentation arises within it not to cause behaviour but to regulate it, direct it, and improve its efficiency. Conscious emotive experience reinforces the action system with additional driving power, and in proportion as intelligence guides the direction taken in its expression, the efficiency of the behaviour is improved. In both embryological and phylogenetic development, intrinsically activated motility precedes reaction to external stimulation. The body acts before it reacts. In embryo-genesis myogenic movement precedes neurogenic action. Muscles can act and react before they have any nervous connections. In the light of these findings the Tantric conception of an embryo's development, as intrinsically connected with motility in its various forms and movement along certain pathways, is less fantastic than the wording makes it appear.'

Judson C. Herrick makes another significant statement which may perhaps help to explain Tantric ideas. He says: 'Mind emerges from the non-mental, and it may in turn control not only the behaviour of the body but also its structural organization. It is recognized by everybody that disorder of bodily structure may disturb the mind. The converse is equally evident, as painfully illustrated by the prevalence of gastric ulcer associated with chronic anxiety or worry. Equally striking changes in the physical structure of bodily tissue and its chemical processes have been induced by hypnotic suggestion. The ulcers or hypnotically induced blisters are not caused by a non-physical entity called a mind but by a psycho-neural bodily process that is organically related with the other vital functions.' In the Tantric texts this is what is called 'creative potentiality' (thig-le), certainly not a mind in our sense, which is the end-phase of a long evolutionary process. Neither is it physical, although it becomes observable only in the physical organization commonly called a body. It is a unitary principle that may be viewed either as structure or as motility, or as the controlling and structuring process. Conversely it is group-patterned by the carry-over of experience traces or as C.D. Broad more exactly calls them 'experientially initiated potentialities of experience'. The same author cautiously advances a theory which is a corner-stone in Tantrism. He says: 'We must therefore consider seriously the possibility that each person's experiences initiate more or less permanent modifications of structure or process in something which is neither his mind nor his brain. There is no reason to suppose that this substratum would be anything to which possessive adjectives, such as "mine" and "yours" and "his" could properly be applied, as they can be to minds and to animated bodies . . . [but] . . . as we know nothing about the intrinsic nature of the experientially initiated potentialities of experience, we cannot say anything definite about the intrinsic nature of the common substratum of which we have assumed them to be modifications. As there is no reason whatever to think that such potentialities of experience are, or could be, themselves experiences, there is no reason whatever to suppose that the substratum is a mind. On the other hand, it could hardly be any particular body. It does not seem impossible that it should be some kind of extended pervasive medium, capable of receiving and retaining modifications of local structure or internal motion'. All this puts a new interpretation on the word 'creative'. In this context its meaning is not that of an act of construction, since it is neither wholly active nor wholly passive. It is rather best described as 'responsiveness.'*

Just as the pathways linked man with something greater than himself, so also motility is not restricted to his limited existence but shares in a wider context. This is indicated by the reference to the vibratory rate in relation to the houses or signs

* rlung — Wind

of the zodiac, which operates in connection with the motor activity of the body when the cusps are reached. In other words our conscious life, which has a strongly conative character, is constantly, though mostly imperceptibly fed by what defies determination and only figuratively is expressed in terms of astrology, or hinted at by the highly technical term 'awareness-motility'.

The creative potentiality can be viewed from various angles, either with relation to the pathways and motility as the structuring and controlling process, or as the presence of something spiritual in man. The use of the words 'spiritual' and 'spirituality' does not imply any sort of so-called 'spiritualism'. I understand these words merely as working concepts, indexes. There is thus a close resemblance to the use of this word by Noel Jaquin who declares: 'I do not wish to use the word "spiritual" in this connexion in any religious or mystic sense, but rather as implying that part of man's being which is a directive counterpart of his physical being in terms of a higher-dimensional existence. This means that our approach to the continued examination of the physical structure and its activities must be made with a full awareness of these unexplored possibilities'.

The Cosmological Interpretations of Sutherland and Still

The same hypothesis in Tantric Buddhist philosophy and the extra dimension – the spiritual element – is in accordance with Sutherland's experience and his references to Dr Still's visionary abilities. For example, the second precept of Still – 'the Rule of the Artery is supreme' – refers to the overall importance of the physical circulatory system as a whole and particularly the vaso-motor system, arteries, veins, lymphatic vessels, body-fluids generally, including the CSF (Cerebro-spinal fluid) which according to Sutherland[5] is 'in command', and therefore of primordial importance, not just in a physical sense. As he points out, the rhythmic fluctuation of the CSF is a motion like that of the tide of the ocean, motivated 'by the same Intelligence that governs the tide of the ocean, governs the rotation of the earth, the sun, the moon and all the planets'. Dr Sutherland mentions the outflow along the nerves and into the lymphatics of what Dr Still mystically referred to as 'the highest known element in the human body', a transmutation, the unknown 'something', analogous to the 'sap of the tree' – something that contains the 'Breath of Life' – not the breath of air, something invisible but which has the inherent quality of brilliant Light: Liquid Light.[6] What other than the Clear Light of the Void (Shunyata)? He continues: 'If you recognized the real element, the breath of light in the cerebro-spinal fluid, I think you would begin to come closer to the success of Dr Still in his knowledge of the human body'. Dr Sutherland also makes a number of references to the equal importance of space – not only the space between material particles and between and within the physical structures and tissues of the body – but he also gives abstract examples, and says that through the end of a telescope one sees 'endless space'.

Dr Still, when examining a patient, could apparently look right through the person's body and acquire knowledge of the abnormalities, without even resorting to touch. Dr Sutherland emphasizes the difference between *obtaining knowledge rather than information*.[7] One must think osteopathy and not just think osteopathically. Thinking osteopathy means that the osteopath is totally identified, i.e. in complete empathy with his or her patient, they are as one. There is no subject and no object and no observer. In this way because of the total openness of the situation, i.e. by tuning in to the Void, knowledge of the patient's illness and problems easily comes.

Thinking osteopathically on the other hand means merely conceptualizing in terms of 'this' and 'that', in which case practitioner and patient are not in true empathy. Granted the more skilled and resourceful be the osteopath in the intellectual exercise of his or her calling, there is virtually no limit to the amount of available objective information, in terms of modern scientific and especially computerized medicine. Fine, but the knowledge obtained can at the best, in terms of effective osteopathic treatment, only facilitate in mechanistic terms the choice and application of this or that technique as being suitable and indicated for this or that abnormality or condition. This is not to say that such treatment will not necessarily be effective, it can be highly so in terms of quantitative symptomatic relief and even superficial cure. This is admirable and probably what most patients want, but it is unlikely that any profound change or in-depth therapeutic response will occur, leading to a flash of conscious awareness – i.e. a need to 'walk on' and mitigate karmic propensities – such as can potentially take place if there should be total empathy in a Tantric sense between patient and osteopath. 'You pay your money – you takes your choice' says the old adage. Patients will automatically and unconsciously choose their osteopath – the one that they need, to help them at that point in universal and cosmic-time, i.e. in terms of whether he or she 'thinks osteopathy' or rather only 'thinks osteopathically'. There is no pejorative element in this natural process. Dzogchen (The Great Perfection) teaches that 'Everything is perfect just as it is' and, as the Ven. Acharyra Trungpa Rinpoche has said, things happen and continue to happen – 'apparently by chance'.

Returning to the Void. In the living tradition of Dr Still, osteopathy is in its fourth developmental phase – the phase of synthesis – the Structure-Function/Function-Structure phase, which is in effect a kind of return to the source, back to the subtle visionary, spiritual, holistic, 'source of things' approach of the Old Doctor,[8] as he has been affectionately called. This is where osteopathy is today, on its second round in the evolutionary spiral. Quite apart from the 'thinking, feeling through the tissues' diagnostic approach, the same principle applies in osteopathic technique whether it is applied primarily in a structural and mechanical sense, or on the contrary in a partial or even totally functional way. By mind-awareness, one 'empties' the mind, ratiocination is suspended and the manual procedure is spontaneously applied with specific therapeutic intent; whether it be a brief or prolonged application, something happens, an event which is as subtle and on the same level as the mysterious 'highest known element' of Dr Still – the level of the Void. There is a kind of transmutation, analogous to that which happens in another context, i.e. in Zen Martial Arts, and indeed in the Tao.

During cranial osteopathic treatment, the disturbed and aber-rant cranial impulses and membrane tensions converge, calm down and finally stop. This is called the 'still-point', when all CRI activity ceases and healing, i.e. re-balancing, takes place. When the CRI starts up again all CRI and membrane tensions are normal.

Referring back to Chapter 3 it was stated that health is the proper relationship between the microcosm, which is man, and the macrocosm, which is the Universe.[9] Disease is a disruption of this relationship. 'Unimpeded reaction of the macrocosm to such a disruption results in a cure, unless the disruption is irreversible when death becomes the cure.' In macro/microcosmic terms the spinal column (including the pelvis) represents Mount Meru, the axial centre of the Universe. Osteopathic somatic-dysfunctions or 'lesions' occur principally at this level when the dynamic homeostatic equilibrium is interrupted, the somatic-dysfunction being the focal point of the break in the time-space continuum. Homeostatic equilibrium is understood in its widest sense, 'horizontally' and 'vertically', both internally within the human organism and externally in its relationship with the immediate and greater environment, even in macrocosmic terms. These interruptions of dynamic homeostatic equilibrium within the human organism manifest on the spinal level in identifiable patterns of somatic dysfunction or 'lesion complexes', each with their primary and secondary somatic-dysfunctions.

There is no permanent 'fixity' in these patterns; such 'fixity' as there is, is invariably determined by the adaptation and compensation and/or pathology present in the dysfunctioning or 'lesioned' area, i.e. in terms of the relative chronicity and the biotypology of the clinical subject concerned and whether or not the causative factors are or have been single or multiple. Even the primary somatic-dysfunction or 'lesion' is subject to the same processes of change.

As mentioned previously, osteopaths are trained in general medicine and make use of all the usual Western medical methods of diagnosis, including X-Rays and Laboratory Tests. In addition, osteopathic diagnosis is just as totally holistic and specific as Tibetan medicine. Its objective is the pin-pointing of the primary and secondary somatic dysfunction complexes in a similarly specific and holistic sense. Relevant to all that has been said, osteopathic treatment employs equally holistic and specific procedures within a fluid and changing clinical context (no two patients' somatic-dysfunction complexes are ever the same). It seeks to correct these and restore the dynamic homeostatic equilibrium on all levels, thus facilitating cure (self-cure in fact) to take place.

The therapeutic intent of osteopathic treatment so applied on this level is analogous to the 'uninterrupted reaction of the macrocosm' in thus reversing the disruption between itself and the microcosm, in this instance, the patient. Moreover, it follows that an increasing ability of the osteopath to put his or her mind into the tissues (as Still did in 'looking right through the patient' – or reaching through to the level of the Essence in Tantric terms)[10] will increase the efficacy of the treatment. Healing under these circumstances takes place at the most fundamental level.

Both Still (the founder) and Sutherland were as many others today still are, osteopaths not solely operating on a three-dimensional mechanistic plane, especially in this fourth phase or decade of osteopathy. This connotes in both diagnosis and treatment, an additional, not substitutional, multi-dimensional approach with higher levels of the mind involved and in control. This approach allows for much more than the purely material objective reality upon which the views and concepts of the anatomy, physiology, biochemistry, etc., of Western medicines are based. It therefore follows that osteopaths so 'tuned in' are not solely manipulating and influencing the gross structures of the Outer Form, i.e. the purely physical anatomy (structure) and physiology (function), but also the Inner Form.

Indeed the Inner Form is also influenced – the cakras (khorlo), the nadis (rtsa), prana (rLung), the humours (nēs-pa or nyes-pa) and the cosmic-physical energies are described in the Tantric texts of Tibetan Buddhism at the level, as Dr A.T. Still said, of the 'highest known element in the human body'. It is here that the diagnostic methods of Tibetan medicine, the examination of the pulses and urine plus palpation of the spinous processes and other reflex areas peripherally, as a means of directly assessing the imbalance of the Three Humours and other clinical relevancies can blend in and complement osteopathic diagnostic procedures.

The meeting point between evolving osteopathic concepts within a Western context and, on the other hand, Tibetan medicine which represents an intrinsically Eastern viewpoint based as it is on the Buddhist Tantras, is thus in evidence.

16

Osteopathy III

Body-Mind Relationships: Similar Ancient and Modern Views

It is recognized in Tantric Buddhism that although mind-development is of over-riding importance, a person cannot hope to attain the highest mental and spiritual levels by this means alone. Yantra Yoga emphasizes this implicitly – there is clear instruction that it is absolutely essential to develop physical bliss and health before any attempt is made to pursue any mental or spiritual development. Physical body-balance must be achieved first, and, moreover, the importance of the physical is constantly stressed in relation to the mind and human experience. This principle is seen operating at the deepest levels of Buddhist thought and psychology.

The body as mentioned previously is seen as the composition of the Five Elements. Simply re-stated:

Earth – provides the structure and mass from which the mind can operate at both a gross and subtle level.
Water – allows growth to take place.
Fire – activates metabolism.
Air – provides for growth and development.
Space – gives room to exist.

Each of the elements are interrelated from the grossest to the most subtle levels. The latter exist as energy channels and pathways or Inner Form which sustains function for the Three

Humours of Wind, Bile and Phlegm. The former manifest as the outer, physical form, i.e. the gross structure.

rLung (Wind) – is responsible for all voluntary and involuntary functions of the body.

Bile – is responsible for all secretory functions.

Phlegm – is concerned with all digestive functions.

Function therefore operates and belongs to the subtle level of the body. At the most subtle level the life-sustaining Wind operates. This is located around the heart and it flows through the life-sustaining wind channel. This particular energy is that which sustains the Pure Mind – the mind that travels from one lifetime to another.

To re-cap, it is a basic Buddhist belief that no state of consciousness can operate at any level without energy (Wind) which has moreover a physical basis. This way of thinking and understanding is basic in Tantric medicine and, equally, in using any somatic approach in treatment. It is accepted that the state of the body does affect the state of the mind, body and mind being interdependent. Body can affect mind and mind can equally affect body. Indeed the Tibetan understanding of the processes con- cerned is virtually identical with the osteopathic concept of somatic-dysfunction. In the teaching in osteopathic principle given in the European School of Osteopathy, somatic-dysfunctions are described as somatico-somatic, somatico-visceral and somatico-psychic and conversely psycho-somatic and viscero- somatic.

In the West, we are inclined to think that many concepts, including psycho-somatics, are solely the product of modern discovery, when in fact they have existed in the East for hundreds of years, as for instance in ancient Buddhist thinking. Tantric Buddhist medicine believes that a counterpart of the personality also exists physically. Recognition of this, however, does not negate the importance of the mind in Buddhist thinking. Tibetan physicians have over the centuries spent much time studying body-structure, its movements and muscular activities, its energy-patterns and rhythms inasmuch as they pertain to the purely physical and organic aspects as well as the functional levels. This eventually led to the adoption of the concept of the Three Humours. While appreciating the importance of the physical body as such, they realized also that there was much more than just mere body-structure itself. Ancient yogi physicians were well aware of how the part affects the whole and vice versa, and of the functional rapport between systems and organs and disturbances of structure, and how these can relate to disease processes.

Touch-Sensitivity Diagnostic Technique

In order to monitor functional reactions of the internal organs, inasmuch as they may be affected by diet and behavioural patterns, it was necessary to find some way of assessing these. It seemed logical to study the functional behaviour of the body as a whole, in relation to specific organ function. This was done principally, sufficient sensitivity permitting, by pulse diagnosis, plus palpation. Tibetan physicians talk of sensitivity of touch to factors other than purely physical – for example, the possibility of interpreting changes of energy levels and the variations in mental/emotional tonus and other subtle dysfunctions. This stresses the importance of being able to actually feel the energy rhythm as it flows through the muscular-structures, i.e. with an appreciation of movement and tension. Tibetan physicians are therefore trained to be highly sensitive, and particularly require sensitive hands. It is recommended that they avoid all activities and factors that would roughen the hands.

All these ancient attitudes and practices are so analogous and basic to the principles and practice of osteopathy which, as a system of medicine, is hardly a mere century and a few years old. Be that as it may, it is still exciting to realize that touch-sensitivity as practised for centuries by Tibetan physicians, i.e. the technique of feeling through the physical even to the mental-energy level, is almost identical with the subtle palpatory method used by contemporary osteopaths.

The Importance of Postural Integrity in Tantric Buddhist Medicine

Bearing in mind the enormous emphasis given in osteopathic practice to postural and weight-bearing integrity it is interesting to see what Tibetan medicine says on the subject. Remembering, too, what has already been said apropos of body-mind relationships, it follows that postural integrity is for Tibetans an integral factor in both medicine and religion. Physical posture is an outward reflection of both behaviour and personality – hence the importance of Yoga. In Tantric Buddhist practice posture equates with mudra, one of the three attributes which relate to body, speech and mind – mudra, mantra and visualization technique, respectively. On the basis that changes in body-posture can modify thought-patterns, then mudra as such relates directly to spiritual metamorphosis. In Tantra the physical body is the person. The implication follows that in order to change the person one must first change the body and thus seek to integrate the physical, emotional, intellectual and spiritual aspects as a whole. At the Tantric level it is not just a question of altering the mind as taught and practised in other Buddhist schools. Tantra goes further than that inasmuch as it says that no change can take place in the mind that does not have its physical counterpart.

To re-cap, on the functional level mental states must depend on physical states even at a gross level, hence the over-riding importance of postural-integrity as expressed in mudra. In Chapter 19 this aspect is dealt with in some detail and in a practical self-help way.

The Difference between Treating and Healing (Dr Lobsang Rapgay's view)

In order for healing to be effective it must involve physical change and growth; therefore these processes must be present during treatment, i.e. if healing is to take place. Not all treatment necessarily brings about change or growth at the time it is given. Real healing should encourage change and growth during treatment. This is the difference between healing and mere treatment. (The depth of clinical response is also mentioned in Chapter 2 in relation to the Essence level.)

The Role of Trauma

The role of trauma in osteopathic etiology is of prime importance, it being one of the principal factors in the cause and evolution of somatic-dysfunctions (osteopathic-lesions). The Tibetan medical view is interesting and integrative with osteopathic thinking on the subject. Trauma, Dr Rapgay explains, throws energy-patterns out of balance, they become totally abnormal. Homeostasis re-adjusts as much as it can, but a return to normal does not always occur. One assumes that he is referring to accidents or macrotraumata.

An interesting example from a Tibetan medical viewpoint was given which demonstrates identical thinking on a common clinical problem and which has its counterpart explanation in osteopathic medicine — that of a so-called allergy to certain foods which was non-existent before the person was subjected to trauma. As Dr Rapgay says — if trauma had affected the 8th/9th dorsal vertebrae, a person who normally did not suffer with any problem of liver and/or gall-bladder function, might in consequence start to find difficulty with so-called 'liverish' foods. But, as he says, this would only be because of the trauma, and the disturbance would therefore be purely functional. In osteopathic terms the trauma would have 'facilitated' D8 and 9 thus producing a 'somatico-visceral' dysfunction (or 'lesion').

Diagnosis of Stress

Within this context there are two principal origins of the 'stress' reaction — mechanical and postural strains (microtraumata) and mental/emotional, i.e. anxiety and other pressures. The Tibetan medical method for diagnosing and evaluating the presence of stress, or the severity of the stress-reaction is fascinating for osteopaths inasmuch as the criterion is simply in terms of the

Table 10 Vertebral enumeration

Tibetan Medicine	Western Medicine
1st Vertebra	7th Cervical Vertebra
2nd Vertebra	1st Dorsal (or Thoracic) Vertebra
3rd Vertebra	2nd Dorsal (or Thoracic) Vertebra
4th Vertebra	3rd Dorsal (or Thoracic) Vertebra
5th Vertebra	4th Dorsal (or Thoracic) Vertebra
6th Vertebra	5th Dorsal (or Thoracic) Vertebra
7th Vertebra	6th Dorsal (or Thoracic) Vertebra
8th Vertebra	7th Dorsal (or Thoracic) Vertebra
9th Vertebra	8th Dorsal (or Thoracic) Vertebra
10th Vertebra	9th Dorsal (or Thoracic) Vertebra
11th Vertebra	10th Dorsal (or Thoracic) Vertebra
12th Vertebra	11th Dorsal (or Thoracic) Vertebra
13th Vertebra	12th Dorsal (or Thoracic) Vertebra
14th Vertebra etc.	1st Lumbar Vertebra etc.

degree of vertebral 'facilitation' present, which is elicited by manual pressure on certain reflex-points and concerned structures.

First of all the points in question are Wind-points. The common or general Wind point on the spine is CVII, but the ATLAS (Suboccipital point) and DIV/V are also important. The crown point situated in the vertex of the head is of primary importance, also those associated with the six fontanellae, and the centre of the palms of the hands and soles of the feet.

For diagnostic purposes when stress is present pressure on any of these points can cause pain – this particularly applies to CVII, DIV/V and the sternal point. If little or no pain is elicited the anxiety or stress level is superficial. If there is great sensitivity it means that the stress reaction on the mental level is already affecting the physical body. An excessive increase in the Wind humour activity can cause the energy to find another outlet (the

Table 11 Spinal and peripheral points

Spinal points	Peripheral points
CVII Common Wind Point	Centre of Sternum (a Chapman's reflex in osteopathy)
CIV/V Common Wind Point	
DI Common Bile Point	Crown Point (vertex)
DII Common Phlegm Point	6 Fontanellae points (parietal) Point on Palms of Hands Point on Sole of Foot

'spill-over' phenomenon of osteopathy). It can overflow into other channels and/or 'energy-blocks' can occur. If the stress reaction problem is primarily resulting in a neurosis, a mild neurosis risks becoming a very severe one or worse.

Pressure is applied to the spinous processes of the vertebrae concerned. In osteopathic terms what has been described is simply the degree of 'facilitation' which is the index of the stress reaction.

It would be helpful and pertinent to see the human spine and musculo-skeletal structures from a Tibetan doctor's point of view. First of all the enumeration of the vertebrae is different, as Table 10 illustrates. The 1st vertebra for the Tibetan is the vertebra-prominens or CVII in occidental anatomy.

Apart from the general or common wind reflex-points found at the level of CVII (1st vertebra) and CIV/V (5th and 6th vertebrae), there are also several peripheral Wind points, as well as common points for the Bile and Phlegm humours, and these are given in Table 11.

Using the patient's own thumb measurement, the Tibetan physician is able to plot cutaneous 'points' which are treated traditionally by heat in the form of moxa and golden-rod therapy (see Chapter 10) and sometimes massage. The treatment is directed to the rlung element (remember rlung (Wind) activates and dominates the activities of all the other humours). Table 12 shows the points on the central channel that are commonly treated in this way, but their osteopathic correspondences and

Table 12 Points traditionally treated by heat

1st Point	which corresponds with the ATLAS vertebra and sub-occipital area and also the vertex of the cranium.
2nd Point	which corresponds with the lower cervical area CVI/CVII.
3rd Point	which corresponds with the upper dorsal area DIII/DIV.
4th Point	the twentieth down from CVII (the 1st vertebra in Tibetan medicine), which corresponds with the sacrum, and is approximately at the level of the sacro-iliac articulations.

connotations in that system of medicine are fundamental.

Osteopaths who are familiar with the Littlejohn-Wernham system of Body-Mechanics, the 'Muscular Chains' (Struyf) and the Cranio-Sacral Mechanism (Sutherland) will realize the close correspondence between these Moxa reflex points and their osteopathic counterparts. It is also interesting that Dr Choedhak emphasizes the importance of treating from above downwards, equally relevant in certain (but not all) osteopathic techniques and approaches. Further, and similar, correspondences with the cakras, spinal-areas, autonomic nervous system and endocrine glands are given in Table 13 (see also Chapter 2).

Dr Lobsang Rapgay, in his Tibetan massage lectures, gave the following specific information regarding certain segmental levels of the spinal column.

DI — This is the Common General Bile Point. Feeling it and being sensitive to tissue changes and energy variations, one is able to detect liver and gall-bladder dysfunctions and also ascertain if Phlegm humour disturbance is involved as well.

DII — This is the General Common Phlegm Point. Similar palpation will give information regarding Phlegm activity.

DIII and — These two segments relate particularly to the lungs
DIV and palpation helps to assess their functional

Table 13 Correspondences between cakras, spinal areas, autonomic nervous system and endocrine glands

Cakra	Spinal area	Autonomic nervous system	Endocrine glands
Crown	Atlas, Axis and CIII	Primarily Parasympathetic (Vagus Nerve)	Pineal and Pituitary
Throat	CVI — CVII	Primarily Sympathetic	Thyroid and Parathyroids
Heart	DII — DIV	Sympathetic	Thymus
Navel	DIV — DIX	Sympathetic	Adrenals
Perineal (Secret Place)	LIII, Sacrum (Lumbo-Sacral and Sacro-iliac articulations)	Primarily Parasympathetic (Sacral outflow)	Gonads

activity. Dr Rapgay describes this also as being the organic site of the Wind humour.

DV — There are two bilateral nerves at this level which join the life-sustaining energy pathways. The energy flow of the life sustaining wind can therefore be monitored by palpation of the energy flow at D5. This is probably one of the most important points because the life sustaining wind is the physical basis for all the mental activities. Dr Rapgay further advises that one should always check this point in neurosis and even psychosis. He also mentioned that, in long meditation retreats, it is at this point evidence that the meditation is wrong will manifest. This is known as srog-rLung. Checking D5 is therefore important to ensure that all is going well on the retreat. Drastic changes in diet will also register a difference in the energy-flow at D5.

DVI — There is a direct link here to the heart. Therefore DVI is often called the Heart Point. The heart is the site where the most subtle mind resides. DVI is again an important point for studying Wind activity in the body. Whenever one is exposed to any Wind causing factors, for example abstinence from flesh foods, cold weather, isolation in a dry, high altitude climate in retreat – check the DVI for energy-flow. In heart disease, functional or organic, heat applied at DVI is helpful especially in the form of moxabustion. (DV, DVI, DVII are therefore the most important points of all in relation to exposure to stress and Wind causing factors. Learning to palpate in this way is an excellent training in touch sensitivity.)

DVII and DVIII – Are directly connected to the liver and gall bladder together. Although these are Bile organs, Wind dominates their function. Treatment therefore which will help to regulate the Wind element will also help in Bile disturbances.

DVIII and DIX – Together are very directly related to the gall bladder and in a very specific way.

DX – The correspondences from DX onwards would appear to follow on in very much the same way as described in classical osteopathy.

LI – There is a vein direct to the kidneys; and

LIII – Is designated as being an important point which is usually involved in the stress syndrome.

Another interesting set of correspondences is found between the general locations of the Three Humours (see Chapter 4) and the Three Unities of A.T. Still:

Unity No. 1: pelvis, lumbar-spine and lower-extremities.
Unity No. 2: cranium, cervical spine, shoulder-girdles and upper extremities.
Unity No. 3: Thorax, dorsal spine and ribs (trunk) viz:

General location of:
  rLung   (Wind)   – in Unity No. 1
  mKhris-pa (Bile)   – in Unity No. 2
  Bad-kan   (Phlegm) – in Unity No. 3

As with osteopathy, where functional disease manifests through somatic-dysfunctions, so Tibetan medicine identifies these with

Wind. Therefore Wind = somatic-dysfunction and Wind energy-flow changes at the segmental spinal level manifest as segmental facilitation.

The Tibetan physician is therefore palpating the functional element of disease in virtually the same way as the osteopathic physician palpates somatic-dysfunction. The treatment of course differs, the Tibetan physician massages the points and/or makes topical applications of herbs, etc., whereas the osteopathic physician adjusts and corrects the somatic-dysfunctions or 'lesions'.

It is very important that the points be selectively and specifically treated, says Dr Rapgay. The same of course applies in osteopathy and particularly in terms of SAT (Specific Adjusting Technique) where it is well understood that unspecific treatment leads to less effective results, i.e. in cases of course where SAT is particularly indicated.

Conclusions

Hopefully enough will have been said to show why osteopathy is, in my opinion, after a study of the similarities and parallels, a perfect complement to Tibetan medicine. Obviously I am biased, firstly as a practising osteopath and a teacher of that discipline – particularly the philosophy, principles and clinical applications – and, secondly, as a practising Buddhist in the Tibetan tradition. For this reason, Chapters 14, 15 and 16 are much longer and more detailed than those dealing with other heterodox systems of medicine. However, interesting and convincing as the intellectual considerations may be, as Sutherland has said – acquiring knowledge is not the same thing as obtaining information.

During my ten weeks' stay in Dharamsala in 1977, with the express purpose of investigating Tibetan medicine, it so fell to my lot that much of my spare time was almost solely taken up in practising osteopathic medicine on the spot, and in the Amchi tradition, without remuneration I should add. Since all of my patients were either monks or very poor Tibetan refugees and life in the Himalayas being what it is, this means that hill people are very subject to a variety of trauma. This factor superimposed on the lower-altitude aspect, to which many Tibetans find difficulty in adapting, indicated to me a certain deficiency in the available medical care in the settlement, not fully covered by either the Tibetan medicine or allopathic faciltiies available. This gap was occupied by patients suffering from a variety of complaints, not by any means solely musculo-skeletal, indeed many functional, all of which had principally a traumatic etiology, either resulting from actual accidents or prolonged physical and/or mental stress. Dr Tenzin Choedhak's views in respect of the latter, something which in its present form was almost unknown in the old Tibet, were mentioned in Chapter 7.

For me, the itinerant osteopath doing my daily rounds of home-visits under the blue skies and warm sun of the Himalayan Spring this was one of the happiest and most rewarding times of my life. The profusion of exotic flowers and birds, the huge rhododendron trees, the mountain goats and white monkeys, these were my constant companions. But this is not all. The great blessing was to be within walking distance of Thekchen Choeling, the seat of His Holiness the 14th Dalai Lama, the living Buddha of our time. I was loth to leave.

General Note

This chapter is a synthesis of material given on Tibetan massage and moxa or moxibustion treatment respectively, by Doctors Lobsang Rapgay and Tenzin Choedhak, interpreted and annotated by the author.

17

Psychological counselling with Buddha Dharma and Tibetan medical philosophy as a basis

Psychological Problems Commonly Experienced in the West

In a Western clinical context the average patient's 'hang-ups', in terms of specific fears and anxieties, would seem to express themselves as follows:

1. Fear of death predominates with fear of old-age and disease [and in males particularly of losing potency] coming second;
2. Fear of change;
3. Fear of losing one's job, income, position in society, partner, etc.;
4. Fear of losing self-esteem, friends and admirers, not being thought well of, etc.;
5. Fear of the unknown.

All these fears, with the short and long-term emotional reactions that they subsequently invoke, give rise to lack of self-confidence, conflict, frustration and insecurity, which creates dukkha in terms of the general unsatisfactoriness of life, if not frank suffering, being the fruits that are our 'hang-ups' and paranoia. This is quite apart from the more established clinical, but still functional, disturbances of the mind; the common neuroses such as hysteria, obsessional and compulsive states, phobias (such as claustrophobia and agoraphobia) and complexes, which may need special handling by competent and suitably qualified psychotherapists. In a Western sense this would mean referral to either a psychiatrist or psychoanalyst, but in a Tantric Buddhist context to a lama.

Apart from specific anxiety-states and the more serious groups of common neuroses, which correspond in terms of 'stress-disease' with Selye's 'specific stress factor' aspect, there is also the problem of the unspecific and undefined anxiety that so many people suffer from, manifesting in a state of constant and excessive tension, 'uptightness' and a fear that 'something terrible is going to happen' – 'l'angoisse' as it is so poignantly described in the French language. This in its turn corresponds with Selye's 'unspecific stress factor' aspect.

Of course it is true, as some Western behaviourists would argue, that our basic drives, principally for survival either in groups or as individuals, are fundamental to our behaviour. As one patient, a sufferer from hypoglycaemia once said, 'I certainly get very irritable and "uptight" if I am hungry or if I haven't had sex.' Primitive, atavistic even, but true, and far worse can happen as we are all aware – indeed the most irrational and anti-social behaviour can certainly result, in some cases, from deprivation of the basic needs and suppression of the basic drives. It is not much good giving people Bibles to eat if they are hungry, as the materialist cynic once said. But surely that is begging the question, for by paradox, in some of the most materially affluent Western societies, aberrant behaviour is at its most common. But this is not a contradiction of terms. Of course everyone needs, and indeed is entitled to, a minimal degree of the material – adequate food, housing, recreation and the usual amenities to satisfy the normal basic drives and maintain them in a dynamic equilibrium with the constant activity of body metabolism and the essential homeo-static mechanisms.

Unfortunately, this ideal situation does not pertain for the majority of human beings. In the majority of Western economies and cultures the means and the potential is there, although frequently wasted. In the so-called Third World the opposite is the case – they exist for the minority only.

But *homo sapiens* can think or at least has that potential. Freewill allows for attitudes of mind to operate as moderating factors, in fact if we have the will, in the most effective and decisive way.

Brillat de Savarin, a distinguished Frenchman, once said 'We are what we eat', a not unsurprising statement coming from a native of a country where sophistication of living and the culinary art has reached an as yet unsurpassed perfection in the history of Western civilization.

Nutritional experts are now, however, questioning the veracity of this rather blanket statement. 'We are what we metabolize' would seem to be the contemporary view, which introduces a quantitative element into what is otherwise a purely qualitative, and only partially true, viewpoint.

Buddhist Precepts as a Basis for Counselling

One thing is certain, however much we try to reduce life-phenomenon down to solely mechanistic equations, in direct proportion so will the health, happiness and general well-being of people diminish. The Buddhist saying, 'May all beings be well and happy', would become a nonsense. Paradoxically, there is never a less empty and more dissatisfied person, than the one who is physically totally full and sated.

We are what we think – mind is everything according to Buddha Dharma. Helping one's patients in this clinical context means asking them to sit quietly, as a prerequisite, and ask themselves, as the Ven. Lama Chime Rinpoche constantly says, 'Who am I, where am I and what am I doing?'. Who is this person and why is he or she unhappy and unwell? Why am I here (at all) and why am I very often having difficulties in relating to society generally, my work, other beings and even to the cosmos? What is the purpose of it all – or perhaps there is no purpose? Why are we born, why do we grow old, why do we get sick and why do we die?

Basic Buddhism tells us that Sakyamuni Siddhartha Gautama, the historical Buddha, asked exactly the same question, over 2500 years ago, as Prince of the Sakyas, on leaving the seclusion and totally artificial and protected environment of His father's palace. He set out on His pilgrimage and spent the first part of His life as a mendicant and wandering ascetic to eventually find the answers to these burning questions under the Bodhi-Tree, in present day Bodh Gaya in India. Here in the full moon of Wesak in May, He attained full Enlightenment and found, not only the answer to these questions, but gained full knowledge of everything in the past, present and future.

Merely reading the story of the Buddha's life or indeed His many previous lives in the *Jataka Tales*[1] can provide, if one is open for its acceptance, one of the biggest therapeutic stimuli for any sick and unhappy being. With more specific regard to the 'hang-ups' and paranoia of Western society, the Buddha's teaching on the Three Signs of Being is paramount, especially in relation to fear. These Three Signs of Being are:

1. Impermanence (Anicca)
2. Suffering (Dukkha)
3. Non-Self (Anatta)

Readers are also referred to the many books which touch directly, some in great detail, on the Buddha's life and teachings. Several (my favourites) are listed in the Bibliography.

1. Impermanence

The Buddha taught that nothing is permanent. All compounded things, objects and beings natural or man-made are in a state of constant change and flux. With the passing of the most split moment in time nothing is exactly as it was that split second before. Everything is constantly in a state of becoming and at the same time is disintegrating and dying. The only thing that is permanent is impermanence.

2. Suffering

Buddha taught the doctrine of the Four Noble Truths concerning:

1. suffering itself;
2. the arising or cause of suffering;
3. the cessation of suffering;
4. the means whereby suffering can be overcome and will cease.

The word *Dukkha* was mentioned earlier on. Dukkha was originally freely translated from the Pali as being – suffering. This is now held as being a somewhat inaccurate translation that fails to convey the real meaning, which is much more than just plain suffering, pain, illness, etc., but has an additional meaning in terms of the 'general unsatisfactoriness of life'. The Buddha taught that all life is Dukkha caused by the Three Poisons. These, it will be remembered, relate to the Three Humours (see Chapter 3).

The Three Poisons are sometimes sub-divided into the Five Poisons, which relate to the Five Jinas (Dhyani Buddhas) and the Five Skandhas, as follows:

1. Ignorance
2. Hatred and aggression
3. Passion – lust
4. Envy
5. Pride – slander.
(See Chapter 2)

3. Non-Self

This, sometimes difficult to understand facet of Buddhist doctrine is most clearly explained by John Walters in his book *Mind Unshaken*:

> The trouble is that every individual tends to regard himself as the centre of the universe and as the one person whose desires must be satisfied. Then no sooner does he feel that one desire is satisfied, then another arises. He also wants to feel a sense of permanence. He even talks of settling down here or there 'for good'. The failure of being able to do anything 'for good' is part of his tragedy. Alas, the man's self itself has no individual permanence. His so-called existence is no more than a process of phenomena. Buddhism divides these phenomena into five aggregates (or skandhas). But none of these separately nor all of them together constitutes an ego-entity; therefore, as far as skandhas are concerned, this is non-existent. These five aggregates are material qualities, feeling, perception, co-ordination (habitual tendencies) and consciousness. Of

course they are constantly changing, grouping and regrouping. Thus the 'ego' or 'self' or 'soul' has no real existence. The 'I' that so many unhappy persons regard as so important is but a constantly changing combination of physical and mental phenomena.[2]

Of course in objective reality an ego and a personality does exist as such, I am Tom Dummer and you are Jo Bloggs, but in terms of the law of impermanence there is nothing permanent, solid or certain in the future for either Tom Dummer or Jo Bloggs.

The doctrine of Anatta is beautifully expressed by the poet William Blake:

> **The Fly**
> Little Fly,
> Thy summer's play
> My thoughtless hand
> Has brush'd away.
>
> Am not I
> A fly like thee?
> Or art not thou
> A man like me?
>
> For I dance,
> And drink, and sing,
> Till some blind hand
> Shall brush my wing.
>
> If thought is life
> And strength and breath,
> And the want
> Of thought is death;
>
> Then am I
> A happy fly,
> If I live
> Or if I die.

Karma and Rebirth

Also pertinent to our subject of counselling is the doctrine of karma and rebirth, which is explained fully by the Wheel of Life and the law of dependent origination. Karma (action) is the expression of cause and effect which operates not only in this lifetime, but from lifetime to lifetime until the state of the enlightened mind is reached. Karma is the continuous stream of energy, the consciousness (essence of the mind) produced by a person's actions and deeds of body, speech and mind in one lifetime, and passes on in unending succession to others. Moreover, it is stated in *The Secret Life and Songs of the Tibetan Lady Yeshe Tsogyal*:

> In short, wheresoever is human emotion, there is sentient life; wheresoever is sentient life, there are five elements, there is space; and insofar as my (Yeshe Tsogyal) compassion is co-extensive with space, it pervades all human emotion.[3]

There is no permanent 'soul entity' in Buddhism which is reincarnated in the sense and understanding of Hinduism, or a soul that goes either to heaven or hell as a final happening, as it is taught in the Christian faith. These are the principal facts of Buddha Dharma that can serve the practitioner well in helping each patient to understand his or her particular Dukkha involvement.

Practical Procedures

In addition, maybe the following notes on practical procedures will prove useful:

1. Advice to the patient

Travelling by train quite recently in an old-fashioned compartment, a perfect medium for graffiti, I was somewhat astonished to perceive the following:

Things that happened in the past
Only happened in your mind
So forget your mind
And you'll be free.

Strong meat to digest while ambling through the Kent countryside on a hot summer's day, but highly practical advice, for most of us find it much easier to live in the past and future rather than do the most obvious and logical thing and live in the present.

All the different aspects of fear outlined above will be found on reflection to be either groundless, or of little consequence, in view of the Teachings inherent in the Three Signs of Being and particularly through an acceptance of the doctrine of karma and rebirth.

The buddha also likened life to the flow of a river. We should flow along with it, mid-stream with full confidence and not get 'hung-up' with all the diversions and side issues, sometimes very seductive, on the banks. To accept this, to put space around oneself, to have confidence and to stop worrying, to go with it, and above all to stop trying to influence events and things – to let them just happen as they surely will, even though the ego won't like it and may send out strong signals that it is not taking kindly at all to the threat to its very existence. This is where meditation can be of assistance.

2. Meditation

The back-bone of Buddhist practice comes to its own in these circumstances. Simple, basic meditation (samatha), will work wonders, not only in terms of quieting the mind as such, but also by the reduction of nervous tension, which can materially help physical disease. The technique is to just sit quietly, watching the breathing, and letting one's thoughts come and go. Regarding meditation, the following extract from a Buddhist journal is of interest:

Chronic pain is diminished in programs such as those employed by Kabat-Zinn at the University of Massachusetts Medical School, in which subjects are taught a technique of mindful meditation. Cholesterol levels in hypercholesterolemic men fall by one-third when they are taught to clear their mind twice daily for a certain period of time. The recurrence rate of heart attack is reduced significantly when persons learn to modify the content of consciousness through learned relaxation. The stability of the heart's rhythm can be positively affected through techniques of meditation. A common feature of these and a myriad of similar studies is that as consciousness is recognized as occupying a valid position in the orderly sequence of events called health or illness, one's health flowers. New patterns emerge. New relationships become recognizable, and health is heightened.

(Dr Larry Dossey, 'Space, Time and Medicine', *Vajradhatu Sun*, September 1983.)

3. Counselling

This is of course combined directly with other advice, particularly in the form of 'behavioural therapy' (see Chapter 8).

Conclusion

In conclusion I quote Terry Clifford:

All the 84,000 defilements which Buddha described can be condensed into these three. The medicine that cures them and their painful effects is the 3-fold training which summarizes the path of Dharma: virtue-compassion cures lust, greed, grasping; contemplation-meditation cures anger, hatred, repulsion; and wisdom-insight cures ignorance and basic confusion. Of these, the development of wisdom (*prajna*) is the most important, for it attacks the root poison, ignorance, from which the others arise. Therefore *prajna* or wisdom is the supreme medicine that cures all diseases and pain.[4]

18

Practising Tibetan medicine in conjunction with Western scientific medicine

In Dharamsala there are two hospitals, the allopathic, i.e. Dharamsala Hospital as such, and the Delek Hospital founded in 1971 by His Holiness the Dalai Lama, plus accommodation for bed-patients in the more recently built annexe of the Tibetan Medical Centre. Thus the population of Dharamsala and district have access to both the orthodox Western system and Tibetan medicine itself, which are complementary to each other. This is also the case in other parts of India where there are Branch Clinics of the Tibetan Medical Institute.

Since Tibetan medicine is a holistic system of medicine and allopathy is not, it would seem more logical to practise it in the West within the context of other systems of holistic medicine, unless by fully and traditionally trained practitioners of Tibetan medicine.

But, is this strictly true or is it not rather 'loading the question'? Any form of medicine or, indeed, any activity come to that, does not practise itself; it of course depends on the human element, the practitioner. Moreover the practitioner has a mind with infinite possibilities, according to Tantric Buddhism. So if we really believe that mind can accomplish all, is it not more a question of attitude of mind? Unfortunately with most of us, our minds and consequently our thinking are so conditioned, particularly by the Three Poisons (sometimes subdivided into Five), that the state of mind of 'seeing things as they really are' (Ven. Acharya Trungpa Rinpoche) is seldom attained, except by the very spiritually advanced and considerably enlightened who have realized 'absolute truth'. For the rest of us, however much we may excel in our logical and sometimes highly complex intellectual manipulation of the 'relative truth' (the concept of 'scientific method' perhaps being the prime example of the century), however clear we may attribute our thinking to be, our ratiocination is still clouded by our prejudices, 'hang-ups' and conditioning – ethnic, cultural, social, political, religious *et al.*

What has all this to do with practising Tibetan medicine within the context of orthodox medical practice? It can be said that the attitude behind the antipathy between the advocates of orthodox and unorthodox medicine, both lay and professional, is a fair runner up to the intolerance, cruelty and consequent human suffering that is caused by certain aspects of religious fanaticism and their counterpart on the level of extremist politics.

Fortunately today, as mentioned elsewhere, there is a distinct change of heart, and co-operation – albeit limited at present – is growing between doctors and qualified medically unregistered practitioners. In the UK, the adoption of the term 'complementary' medicine instead of 'alternative', by most professional non-medically registered holistic medicine practitioners and their professional bodies, has been a positive step forward. This move has contributed enormously by inherent implication that we can if we really want to, co-exist together for the good of all, i.e. as far as any groups of human beings will allow each other to do so.

Personal Responsibility

As with all things, the initiative for change rests with individuals. First of all comes the awareness of the need, the idea germinates and the means whereby develops – i.e. the technique: learning the therapeutic discipline. Then follows the most difficult thing of all – having the moral courage to do it, to take all the risks *vis-à-vis* one's colleagues and friends, that non-conformists always have to take and then as the late Judge Christmas Humphreys continuously said, 'Walk on!'

Within the context of our subject as mentioned above (to be aware of the need, to acquire the means and to have the moral courage to actually do it), there are many doctors who have given up practising allopathic medicine and who have become homoeopaths, acupuncturists or osteopaths instead. I personally know of two who are still practising GPs within the British National Health Service and there may be many more, who have totally reorientated their clinical approach to one of health-building and spiritual counselling, combined with a minimal prescription of allopathic drugs.

First came the awareness of the need for change. Both of these GPs had altered their approach in almost identical ways, i.e. (a) by first of all allocating at least half an hour per session per patient and (b) putting the onus on patients to accept more and more responsibility for their own health.

How does this work in practice? Firstly, half-hour sessions allow for a proper clinical rapport to develop between the doctor and the patient with all the advantages of the old 'family doctor' relationship, somewhat discredited by 'scientific medicine'. Secondly, taking responsibility for one's own health presupposes questioning life-styles that may be unwise or even detrimental to maintaining good health and that may indeed be disease-causing, and being prepared to make a change for the better. Here, the doctor, having acquired the necessary knowledge in terms of the role of 'physician heal thyself', spends the half-hour period in giving advice and help on virtually the same lines as his Tibetan doctor counterpart does in terms of 'behavioural therapy' – a Western version of course – plus general counselling in terms of helping the patient to cope with their emotional and life-situation difficulties.

Both GPs in question happen to be very spiritually motivated in the Christian tradition and therefore such counselling would naturally be orientated accordingly. The mode of medicinal treatment under these circumstances is minimal, by comparison with much of the over-prescription usually associated with allopathic practice.

The Incorporation of Tibetan Medical Principles

Should a regular doctor, or any practitioner come to that, be drawn to the idea of practising Tibetan medicine, acquaintance with Buddhism would be presupposed or indeed initiation and

Dharma practice may even have been adopted. It is suggested that the incorporation of Tibetan medicine principles and practice could be on the following lines:

1. The adoption of the tradition, philosophy and principles based on Buddha Dharma and the Root Tantra.
2. Acquiring skills in Tibetan diagnostic methods in order to particularly appreciate the complex body-mind, mind-body relationships, and to be able to diagnose the humoural basis of the patient's problem.
3. Evolve a very comprehensive and effective approach in behavioural therapy and related counselling.
4. By adopting this totally different approach interpret pharmacognosy and the allopathic Materia Medica accordingly.

Dr Lobsang Rapgay puts it totally in perspective. He says:

Change is inevitable because it is the law of nature for all things to undergo transformation, and this is true of every aspect of existence. And yet in medicine, it would be wishful thinking to even imagine that any system can replace the Western orthodox system of medicine, for after all it is the only system that is universally recognized. At this stage, the scope of systems like the Tibetan one is to identify areas like psychiatry, doctor-patient relationships, the way to care for a patient, treatment and ways to handle terminal patients, and so on, and see how its own traditional methods can be modified to possibly serve as adjunctive methods of therapy in the practice of Western medicine.

('Mind Made Health – a Tibetan perspective', *Vajradhatu Sun*, August/September 1983.)

If allopathically trained physicians are able to successfully change over and practise other forms of holistic medicine, why should they not also practise Tibetan medicine?

19

Self-help through Tibetan Buddhist philosophy and medicine

I was recently struck by the simplicity of presentation of a profound subject in an article which appeared in the *Tibetan Review* June 1985 on 'Tibetan Meditation – A Way of Relaxation' by Tseten Dolkar, a résumé of which will be found further on in this chapter.

The substance of this article has already proved to be of immense value to patients in my own practice, adjunctive to the 'de-stressing' techniques that so many osteopaths employ today in order to help their 'screwed-up' patients. The term 'screwed-up' is in no way meant to be derogatory – it means what it literally says. As so often is the case, the vernacular expresses, in a colourful manner, the current state of the world we live in and the reactions and ultimate state that so many human beings find themselves in, in relation to it. This is often to the detriment of their health, well-being and happiness. Such is the enormity of the problem today, that the effects of stress are no longer confined to human beings. Even domestic animals also suffer their fair share and often become neurotic like their owners.

Osteopaths, through the application of manual techniques, help 'screwed-up' people directly by various 'release' techniques, traditional 'lesion' correction, functional and cranial (see Chapters 13, 14 and 15). Osteopaths of course are not unique in this respect, practitioners of other manual medicines also help their patients similarly. This is fine but often the effect is only too short-lived. Releasing the 'stressed' patient in this way can be most valuable and productive. At least for a point in time there is a release from what otherwise appears to be, especially in an experiential way for the patient, an inexorable, relentless pressure, sometimes continuous day and night, for sleep does not always bring even temporary relief. Sedatives and copious amounts of alcohol may provide a temporary solution but this is usually transient until the next 'fix'.

Fortunately we live at a point in time where 'self-help' is strongly in vogue. At one time patients were not the least disposed to help themselves. Even to persuade the obvious sufferer from, say, the effects of just a simple lack of exercise to make a personal effort was a really big deal. Now the pendulum has certainly swung a great deal in the opposite direction – 'self-help' is now very *much* the order of the day.

Within the context, Tibetan Buddhist philosophy and medicine has much to offer in the West where, because there are few or no Tibetan doctors, help in the direct tradition of Tibetan medicine is almost non-existent. The following suggestions and procedures will, it is hoped, be found to be both practical and useful.

Self-help in the Tibetan Buddhist tradition may be summarized as follows:

1. Procedures and practices directed at helping the mind.
2. General and relevant dietary measures (see Chapters 7 and 9).
3. Consciously altering behavioural-patterns and particularly those related to environment and biological needs (see Chapter 9).
4. Self-medication.

These are grouped together in the following pages, rather than treated as separate topics.

Procedures and Practices Directed at Helping the Mind

Causes of Mental Disturbance

It is important first of all to recall how the mind gets disturbed. First, discursive thinking and ratiocination are not the mind itself but only the function of the mind. What we call mental activity is usually due to some external stimulation, which is not always solely due to non-physical causes. The process involves the Wind humour.

Wind, as Lobsang Rapgay points out, can be increased for instance by a low-protein diet, drinking strong tea and eating light green vegetables, as well as arising from states of anxiety and depression. This can be monitored by assessing the increase of the Wind characteristics by urinalysis. Osteopaths also know that physical trauma can increase Wind activity through disturbance of the spinal mechanisms and postural mechanics generally and particularly through the 'facilitation' of the DIV/V area which is the Wind area in Tibetan medicine (see Chapter 16).

Diet

Self-help in this instance involves attending to diet a priori, i.e. by omitting foods that tend to increase Wind and replacing them by those that diminish the effects of excess Wind. Concerning structural disturbances, where suitable osteopathic care is not available, these can be helped by the techniques of Tibetan massage and/or exercise (Kum Nye for example).

Meditation

Mental relaxation is best achieved by the contemplative process, as Tseten Dolkar clearly advises:

> The common form of meditation used to cope with stress is a simple procedure that can be easily practised by anyone. It involves focusing the mind on physiological processes such as breathing and walking. After obtaining a certain amount of skill with this basic type of meditation, the person shifts to more difficult objects of focus, such as his thought process and emotions. The basic procedure of the technique comes in several steps. The person is required first to choose a comfortable position, which is normally a crossed legged posture known as the lotus position. The Tibetan Buddhists recommend the lotus position since they believe it allows

maximum breathing control and circulation of blood to the limbs of the body. During all sessions the person closes his eyes naturally and without effort to avoid distractions. In order to enhance the quality of meditation, the person initially relaxes the muscles, starting from his feet and progressing up to the calves, thighs and abdomen. Finally the head is loosened, neck and shoulders gently rolled round and the shoulders are shrugged slightly. After completing the preparation, the main part of the meditation comes next. It involves focusing on the breathing process. The person breathes slowly and naturally, wthout forcing the rhythm and during inhalation the attention is focused on the expansion of the abdomen and then on its contraction as he exhales. During the attempts to concentrate on the breath, thought interruptions will inevitably begin to bombard the mind, and distractive images may prevent the person from proper focusing. However, such distractions are not uncommon. In fact, they are natural and occur frequently and the person is taught not to be bothered by them. The way to deal with these interruptions is to learn how to respond to them as casually as possible and bring back the mind on the breath.

Visualization

Wind can also be balanced even more effectively by those versed in the visualization techniques used in Tantric practice, particularly Dzogchen. By visualizing a white letter (Tibetan) AH[1] in the space between the eyes before going to sleep, Wind is automatically balanced up.* The Five Elements can also become similarly imbalanced for physical as well as mental reasons. For example Dr Pema Dorjee[2] has pointed out that in Diabetes Mellitus the Water and Earth Elements are in excess. Obviously, dietetic adjustment is crucial but, as Professor Namkhai Norbu also points out, the Five Elements can be balanced up, again by a similar visualization technique as described for Wind. But instead of visualizing a letter AH between the eyes, a rainbow-coloured

---

* Note: to be effective this advice should only be followed within the context of Professor Namkhai Norbu's instructions generally.

bindu (thig-le) is visualized (the five rainbow colours – red, blue, green, yellow and white correspond with the Five Elements).

Balancing the Five Elements

The 9th Karmapa, Wangchuk Dorje, explains how posturally all five elements can be balanced up – i.e. by sitting correctly in the Vairocana meditation position. This asana, by the way, has an interesting correlation. According to the Matthias Alexander Method the head/body relationship for optimum health and balance is none other than the Vairocana meditation position, it corresponds exactly. One just needs to look at a Buddha image, particularly from the side-view, to see that this is so. His Holiness Wangchuk Dorje[3] describes the process as follows:

Vairocana Asana
The vajra (or lotus) position is being seated on a cushion with both legs crossed, the feet resting on the opposite calves or thighs (or in the crossed leg posture). This position controls the DOWNWARD GOING ENERGY.
In order to place the energy winds of the solid element of the body into the central energy-channel, straighten your spine like the end of a spear. In order to induce the energy-winds of the liquid element into the central channel, place your hands in the equipoise meditation posture* and hold them beneath your navel, and also raise both your shoulders back and even. To induce the energy-winds of the heat element into the central channel, keep your neck slightly bent like a hook. To induce the energy-wind of the gaseous element into the central channel, have your eyes neither wide-open nor shut tight, but gazing at a point straight ahead from the tip of your nose. Your tongue and lips whould be in their normal, relaxed condition or you may have your tongue touch your upper palate.

---

* The equipoise meditation posture of the hands is with them in the lap, palms facing upwards, left hand beneath the right and with the thumbs upright and touching.

Controlling Mind Tonus

In meditation the mind may be:

(a) dull, with a tendency to be drowsy or even to fall asleep. A cool and breezy environment makes for freshness and alertness. Light food also makes the mind light.
(b) agitated, the mind wanders and cannot focus because the meditator is over-excited. It is important to keep warm, do exercise and eat heavy, fatty food.

In order to eliminate:

(a) mental dullness – visualize a white dot at your brow. This will perk you up – the white colour awakens you and your mind naturally becomes brighter.
To calm:
(b) agitation – direct the mind towards a black, lustrous spherical dot the size of a pea which you can visualize at the point in front of you where your folded legs touch your seat.

His Holiness advises that if one has neither mental dullness nor agitation, direct your mind to either a visualized blue dot (or actual blue object) on the ground at a distance at the end of your shadow in front of you. As he further says – 'The blue of a clear, dustless autumn sky is a neutral colour that neither uplifts nor subdues the mind'.

A Self-help Procedure to Help the Mind and Balance Generally: Kum Nye

Tarthang Tulku's introduction to Kum Nye[4] is straight to the point, as this brief quotation from the Preface of Book 1 shows:

Kum Nye relaxation is a gentle healing system which relieves stress, transforms negative patterns, helps us to be more balanced and healthy, and increases our enjoyment and appreciation of life. In these times when confusion and chaos are so much a part of daily activity, we are often too tense and charged up to enjoy life. Kum Nye opens our senses and our hearts so that we feel satisfied and fulfilled, and can appreciate more fully every aspect of our lives. Even in a short time, the quality of experience can be enriched, and our lives grow more harmonious. This unique value of the Kum Nye system of relaxation is that it integrates and balances two approaches, the physical and the psychological. Kum Nye heals both our bodies and minds, bringing their energies together to function calmly and smoothly. Because it leads to the integration of body and mind in all our activities, this relaxation has a vital and lasting quality greater than the feeling of well-being experienced in physical exercise, or even in disciplines such as yoga.

The procedural basis of Kum Nye is first of all an understanding of the theory, massage, sitting, breathing exercises and movement exercises, balancing body, mind and senses, stimulating and transforming energy. Tarthang Tulku's two-volume work on Kum Nye relaxation represents a self-help manual *par excellence* in the Tibetan medical tradition.

A Summary of the Main Self-Help Procedures

Conclusion

Self-help may be thus summarized in terms of:

1. methods of mind-training;
2. dietary measures;
3. consciously changing behavioural patterns; and
4. self-medication.

Point 4 requires further elucidation. First of all, it may be asked — is self-medication necessary, desirable or indeed safe? Well, whatever objection we may have, self-medication is firmly ensconced, as the well-stocked shelves of pharmacies and health-food stores demonstrate everywhere, certainly in the West.

Readers who are interested in this form of self-help are advised to write to The Tibetan Medical Centre in Dharamsala who are prepared to mail all over the world personal orders of the standard formula medicines. Lists of products available and particularly those mentioned in Chapter 7 will be sent on request.

Self-Help and Simple but Effective Help for Others from Meditation on the Medicine Buddha (Men-la)

The Fundamental Principles

According to the Teachings by Dr Trogawa Rinpoche[5] this is a Mahayana form meditation, i.e. from a Sutra point of view, involving the Nirmanakaya level of existence. Taking Refuge in the Three Jewels and being actively committed to the raising of Bodhicitta is traditionally the normal prerequisite to this healing meditation. However, those who have not necessarily taken Buddhist vows but who have the awareness of the altruistic attitude of mind, will also find great benefit in doing the meditation, not only for themselves but especially for other people.

According to Dr Trogawa Rinpoche there are three fundamental aspects to Enlightenment:

(a) *Knowledge – Wisdom of Intrinsic Awareness* – this aspect is space-like, it has no centre or periphery and is infinite.
(b) *Love* – there is great compassion with an enlightened mode of seeing all sentient beings equally.
(c) *Power* (Energy) – in the sense of 'Adisthana' – power to give Refuge to beings. Moreover it is this power or energy that we have to trust and work with.

Procedure

In meditation or the absorptive state of mind one cultivates the ability to visualize – in this case the Medicine Buddha. A photograph of a Thangka or a painting in colour is necessary, in order to familiarize the mind. On the other hand, the Medicine Buddha must not be visualized as a solid form in objective outline. He should appear as insubstantial, transparent and mirror-like, like the reflection of the moon in water. One's accompanying feelings should be of Wisdom, Love and Power combined and one should meditate with a deep devotion and intensity of feeling.

Men-la, as visualized in front of us, has all the characteristics of a Buddha. He has the Power and Intention to benefit all beings. He expresses His compassion through His profound healing ability. He can be visualized above the head of a sick person or above one's own head, as the case may be. When walking, visualize Him on your right as in circumambulation. Before going to sleep, visualize Him on your pillow. When eating, visualize amrita* flowing from Men-la into the food.

If you are treating a patient manually, visualize Men-la in front of you and amrita flowing from your hands into the patient. Visualize Him on the palms of your hands and also a Men-la on each finger-tip. In treating a patient medicinally, visualize amrita flowing into the medicines and giving them the qualities of a panacea. Visualize amrita flowing into oneself from the Medicine Buddha, giving or increasing one's capacity to heal.

In treating:
(a) Hot Diseases – one visualizes radiance and a cooling quality of the amrita.
(b) Cold Diseases – again one visualizes radiance but the amrita should be 'heating'.

When there is evident total disequilibrium, i.e. the humours are chaotic, radiance and amrita should be visualized in equilibrium.

In order to concentrate the vital energies for the purpose of prolonging life, this is done within the context of visualizing the Five Elements as follows:

Flesh is identified with Earth – visualize and identify this with a yellow light.

---

* Amrita – nectar. In this context, healing nectar.

Blood is identified with Water – visualize and identify this with a white light.

Breath – is identified with Wind (Air) – visualize and identify this with a green light.

Body-Heat is identified with Fire – visualize and identify this with a red light.

Consciousness is identified with Space – visualize and identify this with a blue light.

Visualize each light as an emanation radiating from Men-la, which draws out the essence of each of the Five Elements into the Medicine Buddha's bowl, e.g. the essences of Earth, Water, Air, Fire and Space are thus drawn into the bowl. Finally, the mixture of all the Five Elements in Men-la's bowl enters the Crown cakra* of the person, the patient or oneself.

If initiated, recite the Medicine Buddha's mantra with visualization of the Five Lights. All these procedures it is said will lengthen life. You may also dedicate merit – viz. that all beings should reach the Light of the Medicine Buddha and should be heard by Him. The mantra of Men-la, the Medicine Buddha, is:

> TADYATA
>
> OM BEKENTZE, BEKENTZE, MAHA BEKENTZE
>
> RADZA SAMBUGATE SOHA.

The Sutra of The Medicine Buddha**

The Guru of Healing – The Radiance of Lapis
Lazuli, Tathagata
Beduriya Buddha

Thus have I heard: While wandering thru' many lands to convert beings, the Bhagavan arrived at Vaisali. He dwelt under a tree through which music resounded and with him was a huge host of 8,000 Bhikshus, 36,000 BSMsattvas,*** kings, ministers, brahmins, learned Upasakas, the eight kinds of Nagas and other beings, such as kinnaras and the rest. A vast

---

* Aperture of Brahma, Mahamudra Gate.

** Great Merit for those caring for the sick, also for the sick person, from either hearing or reading this sutra.

*** Bodhisattva Mahasattvas.

community devotedly surrounded him. He taught them Dharma.

Then Manjushri, the crown Prince of the Dharma realm rose from his seat, a thought of the Buddha spontaneously arising in him. He bared his shoulder, bent his right knee to the ground in the direction of the Bhagavan, bowed, joined the palms of his hands and reverently said, 'World honoured one we wish to hear the names of the Buddhas, the particular blessing and the vow made by each of them in former days, in order that hearers may throw off the fetters of Karma to the benefit and joy of beings who live in the period of decline'.

Then the Buddha praised Manjushri saying, 'Good, good Manjushri, out of great compassion you ask me to tell the names of the Buddhas and the blessings of their vows in order to free beings living in the age of decline of the Dharma, from the fetters of Karma which bind them to be of service to them and make them happy. Now listen well and bear in mind what I say. Manjushri said, 'Speak, if such is your wish we are glad to listen'.

Then the Buddha said to Manjushri, 'Eastward from here beyond numerous Buddha realms, there is a world called "As pure as Lapis Lazuli". Its Buddha is called the Lord of Healing, the Tathagata of Azure Radiance, perfectly enlightened, perfect in mind and deed, finder of the way, knower of the world, trainer of men as a skilful charioteer controls his horses, teacher of Gods and men, Buddha, Bhagavan. Manjushri, this world honoured one on becoming a Bodhisattva, made twelve great vows to grant beings their most earnest wishes, thus:

1. I vow that after I have been born into the world and have attained perfect enlightenment, my body shining like a brilliant flame, throwing beams on infinite, countless, boundless worlds, adorned with the 32 major and 80 minor marks of a great man, I will make all beings equal to me.

2. I vow that after I have attained perfect enlightenment, my body shining like Lapis Lazuli, in spotless virtue within and without, in the majesty of its virtue, sitting serenely, adorned with rays brighter than the sun and moon, I shall by my presence inspire understanding of being lost in the

darkness of ignorance, in order that they may act freely.

3. I vow that after I have attained perfect enlightenment, I shall grant to all beings by means of infinite boundless wisdom, the cessation of all their poverty. They shall never lack the things they need.

4. I vow that after I have attained perfect enlightenment, I will bring to the Mahayana those beings who have gone astray and those travelling along the Sravaka and Pratyakabuddha yanas.

5. I vow that after I have attained perfect enlightenment, I shall lead innumerable beings practising moral conduct to attain this conduct in its purity. If they relapse they will become pure again when they hear my name, and will not fall into the three lower realms.

6. I vow that after I have attained perfect enlightenment, beings, mentally or physically defective, shall all be restored when they hear my name.

7. I vow that after I have attained perfect enlightenment, beings tormented by disease, shall, on hearing my name be freed from disease and restored.

8. I vow that after I have attained perfect enlightenment, women tormented by the 100 sufferings of women, shall in the end attain perfect enlightenment.

9. I vow that after I have attained perfect enlightenment, I shall cause all beings to escape the nets of Mara and the fetters of wrong view. If they have fallen into the dense forests of perverted concepts, I shall lead them to the Dharma and gradually induce them to lead the life of a Bodhisattva. Soon they will attain perfect enlightenment.

10. I vow that after I have attained perfect enlightenment, all who are prisoners, sufferers of violence and outrage, shall when they hear my name be freed of their torment.

11. I vow that after I have attained perfect enlightenment, those who commit unskilful acts because of suffering hunger and thirst, shall if they remember my name, be filled. I shall let them taste the Dharma and be perfectly happy and relieved.

12. I vow that after I have attained perfect enlightenment, all without clothes, afflicted by insects, heat and cold, when

they hear my name, remember and cherish it, shall receive
clothing and all their needs be fulfilled.

Manjushri these are the 12 wonderful sublime vows of the
world honoured one, Lord of Healing, the Tathagata of
Azure Radiance, the perfectly enlightened one. These vows
he made when he was a bodhisattva. Furthermore if I
wished to speak of these vows and the ornaments of his
Buddha Realm, for a kalpa or longer, I should never end.
This Buddha land is eternally pure. The ground is of Lapis
Lazuli and all the structures are made of the same precious
substance.

In all respects it is the same as the pure land of Amitabha,
Sukhavati. There are two BSMsattvas* there, the radiance of the
sun and Moon. They are the chiefs of a countless host of
Bodhisattvas. Therefore Manjushri, when this Lord of Healing,
the Tathagata of Azure Radiance, had attained perfect
enlightenment, he saw all beings suffering from disease and
entered into a great Samadhi called 'the removal of suffering
from all beings'. While in this samadhi, a great light shone from
his forehead, and he pronounced the great Dharani:
NAMO BHAGAVATE BHAISHAJA GURU – VAIDURYA PRABHA
– RAJAYA TATHAGATAYA ARHATE SAMYAKSAMBUDDHAYA
TADYA ATHA OM BHAISHAJYE BHAISHAJYE SAMUDGATE
SVAHA. When he in his radiance had spoken this Dharani, the
whole universe was shaken and emitted a great light. All beings
were delivered from disease and misery and attained rest and
supreme happiness.

---

* Bodhisattva Mahasattvas

20

Conclusions and perspective for the future

In a general statement by His Holiness The Dalai Lama on the 23rd Anniversary of the Tibetan National Uprising, the following excerpt is pertinent:

> In any society, the distinction between truth and falsehood, benefit and harm, is ultimately revealed by time and history. Similarly, the actual history of these last twenty three years has done a big summing up of whatever was the truth and whatever the false in the Issue of Tibet. Without resorting to untruth and lies, without fabricating non-existing accomplishments or belittling past achievements and erasing their traces, it is important to apply the reasonable method of 'seeking truth from facts' in analysing and learning lessons derived from a calm and objective study of the roots of right and wrong as they have been revealed and are being revealed by actual history.
>
> At this moment, questions of the old and the new social systems, religion, differing ideologies and systems spring to the mind of many Tibetans in and outside Tibet. As I have mentioned many times before, on this question the Tibetans will have to keep pace with the progressive changes that are occurring in the 20th century world and move towards democratic revolution. The old social system will never be resurrected. The teachings of the Buddha, as contained in the Tripitikas (the three baskets) and the three higher trainings, are beneficial to society since they are based on sound reason and actual experience. These we must preserve and promote.

Difficulties facing Tibetan Medicine in the West

The Vajrayana is the particular form of Buddha Dharma tradition-ally practised in Tibet and Mongolia since the ninth century. It would seem that at the present time, and certainly in the foreseeable future, Tibetan medicine is likely to be equally dependent, both for its survival and future development, on the West and/or outside of Tibet itself. Granted, there are some 5000 monasteries in the Himalayas this side of the Tibetan border and elsewhere in India. On the other hand, there are only some 100,000 Tibetans in exile, not counting those who were resident in Nepal and the other Himalayan kingdoms and Northern India, in Kalimpong for example, before the total Chinese occupation of Tibet in 1959. In addition, there are few more than twenty fully qualified Tibetan doctors (amchis) outside of Tibet proper and these are all practising within the Indian sub-continent. Moreover, it is not possible to ascertain how many have survived and are still practising in Tibet itself. Conversely, the Vajrayana has already spread its influence enormously in the West and the occident generally. There are literally hundreds of Dharma Centres both in Europe and the USA with more high lamas and teachers more readily and consistently available than in India and Nepal for example, and more recently in other countries, notably Australia and South Africa. So while the situation in India is rather one of patiently surviving in exile, largely in terms of preserving and maintaining what remains of Tibetan culture generally, a positive phase of expansion and consolidation of Tibetan culture and Buddha Dharma is taking place elsewhere.

Tibetan medicine, particularly in a practical and clinical sense, has to date unfortunately, for many and diverse reasons, failed to make progress or gain much acceptance in the West. Some of the difficulties may be summarized as follows:

1. These would seem to be arising from fundamental differ-ences in outlook and attitude between East and West generally. Whilst admittedly less rigid and divided than they were, these differing attitudes nevertheless present impor-tant barriers to understanding.

2. Western 'scientific' medicine seems to get particularly 'hung-up' over the religious basis of Eastern medicines. It is acceptable to subject medicinal plants and other remedies and methods to biochemical analysis, etc., but it must stop at that – the mumbo-jumbo is just not on! By paradox, this has been exactly the attitude of Chinese dialectical-materialists: take out what is of value and discard the rest – but who decides what is valuable and by what criteria? Attitudes such as these are in fact a major element in the problem of relating Tibetan medicine to the West.

3. Western medicine is primarily mechanistic and fragmentary in its approach, while Eastern medicine is primarily 'holistic' – e.g. Ayurvedic, Tibetan and Chinese. Nevertheless, some forms of Western medicine, i.e. osteopathy and homoeopathy are also 'holistic', so it is perhaps easier for practitioners of these disciplines to communicate with Eastern practitioners.

4. Although the Western preoccupation with intellectualizing and categorizing as a purely academic study may be satisfactory to many subjects, particularly those of a purely abstract character, neither the Dharma itself (which needs to be practised as well as being read and studied), nor its form of Tibetan medicine with its full clinical connotations, is amenable to this approach.

Essential Differences between Eastern and Western Systems of Medicine

The essential difference at this point in time between Western and Eastern systems of medicine (and this can be said of culture generally) is that in the former religion, philosophy, medicine and indeed politics, now exist as separate entitites. They are no longer essential and inter-dependent parts of a whole closely-knit hierarchical system where the spiritual and temporal organization of society is as one. Such a situation pertained in Europe in the Middle Ages and, until 1959, similarly existed in Tibet. Tibetan medicine, it is argued, being indivisible from Buddha Dharma, i.e. religion, connotes in many Western minds (and especially those concerned with 'scientific' medicine), an esoteric and meta-physical basis and therefore is unacceptable. Here the Dharma is not alone – Chinese acupuncture more recently has suffered similar criticism because of its Taoist basis. Homoeopathy, and even osteopathy in the early days, was subject to the same objection – the latter because its founder was an evangelical Christian. But is this criticism valid? First of all, let us turn to the perennial question – is Buddhism a religion or a philosophy?

As Herbert Guenther points out, the Vajrayana or Tantric Buddhism indigenous particularly to Tibet, and not to be confused at all with Hindu Tantra, is neither or both.

Tantrism is founded on practice and on an intimate personal experience of reality, of which traditional religions and philosophies have given mere and emotional or intellectual descriptions, and for Tantrism reality is the ever-present task of man to be. The critical references to Western ideas, assumptions and conclusions are not meant as a disparagement, but as a means to highlight the contrast between two divergent conceptual frameworks, the one, predominantly mechanical and theistically nomothetic; the other basically dynamic and existentially appreciative. (Herbert Guenther, *The Tantric Way of Life*, Shambhala Publications Inc.)

To emphasise these differences would serve no useful purpose, but to be aware of them is necessary, since understanding Tibetan medicine is likely to be difficult if one approaches the subject with a this or that approach. Herbert Guenther's chapter 'The Problem of Translating Texts' in his book *The Life and Teachings of Naropa* (OUP, 1963) is very clear and helpful to this end.

Problems from a Western Viewpoint

Let us therefore examine a few of the possible aspects and topics to be found in Tibetan medicine that are liable to make Western eyebrows rise, e.g. deities, peaceful and wrathful, the ubiquitous Tantric Buddhist symbolism, the importance given to mantras, possession by evil spirits as an important cause of illness, karma – the very antithesis of the Cartesian logical view of the world, or so it would seem.

Some Modern Philosophical Approaches

Lama Govinda, in *Foundations of Tibetan Mysticism* goes as far as saying that the Buddha was a 'free-thinker'. Certainly, Sakyamuni Buddha – the historical Buddha – in the Judaeo-Christian sense was no god, only a man, albeit an extraordinarily enlightened man. Moreover, Buddhism teaches in an ontological sense that there is no creation, no beginning and no end. All life and living processes are in a constant state of flux and change and permanence, as expressed by cycle, rhythm and periodicity – on all levels life is perpetuated and self-motivating. This is explained in biological terms (Western) by Alan Watts in his prefatory essay to *Outlines of Mahayana Buddhism* by D.T. Suzuki (Schocken Books, New York, 1967) in his references to Dewey's theory of the transitional nature of the relationship between the individual and the world, i.e. organism and environment existing as one 'steady state system' which is postulated as an alternative to the 'vitalist' theory of life.* As Alan Watts says (page xxii):

> Thus as Western science approaches a view of the world as a unified field of behaviour, it approaches an idea of the Dharmakaya, the Universal Body (organism), or the Dharmadhatu, the Universal Field.

Such views of life and the world we live in are identical with the very core of Buddhism and are not contradictory. Timeless existence, not inconsistent with theories of evolution, astronomy and space exploration, is expressed in *The Threefield Lotus Sutra* (Weatherill/Kosei, New York/Tokyo, 1975). In reference to a future Buddha it reads: 'That Buddha will make (his) buddha-land of a three-thousand-great thousand fold universe (of worlds as many) as the sands of the Ganges...'

Buddhist Symbolism and Carl Jung

Meantime, it may be simply said that Buddhist symbolism is a method of communicating meaning that cannot be expressed

* L. Von Bertalanfy, *Problems of Life*, Harper, New York, 1960.

solely by words, leading to a fuller and deeper understanding not normally achieved through purely intellectual means. Buddhism is not the only sphere of human activity or culture that relies on symbolism for its expression and rationale. Carl Jung has made this infinitely clear in his book *Man and His Symbols*. Deities are but symbolic archetypal projections of the Dharmakaya (Universal Mind in Jung's terms) manifesting on the various levels of the human mind. Images are objectivized artifacts of the spiritual energies represented by this or that deity, and are not pagan objects to which the heathen in their blindness bow down, but simply represent the whole spectrum of human qualities – temperament, character, mental constructions and feeling-tone. Their proper visualization is an essential means of overcoming the negative mental elements either contributing to or accompanying many states of ill health and unhappiness.

The Role of Mantras in Healing

Mantras express the archetypal and fundamental sounds and energies essential to a harmonized balance of the Five Elements, the basic stuff of the universe, and consequently, the Three Humours in relation to the psychic channels and centres. Their role and potential therapeutic value, as with prayer generally, is very real, in both the restoration and maintenance of health.

Possession by Spirit Entities as a Cause of Disease

Possession by spirit entities as a cause of mental disease is certainly not totally rejected in Western psychiatric circles, especially concerning distinct personality changes and other psychotic manifestations, and is certainly not rejected by the Christian Church. Karma reflects the law of cause and effect which is not totally unknown and/or unacceptable in the West!

Conclusions

Concerning a perspective for the future, as previously mentioned there are two distinct possibilities which allow for a parallel course of action and as such are not necessarily independent of each other – in fact quite the opposite is the case.

1. (a) The continued preservation of the unbroken lineage of traditional Tibetan medical teaching and practice, in terms of what is being done by the Tibetan Medical Centre in Dharamsala, and also by Doctors Yeshi Donden, Lobsang Dolma, Ven. Trogawa Rinpoche and the other amchis outside of Tibet.

   (b) To preserve as far as possible what written knowledge of Tibetan medicine there is already in existence outside Tibet, both that which is still untranslated from the Tibetan and Mongolian texts and that which is already translated into European languages.

   (c) In this respect, the important translation work, into English, which is currently being carried out in India at the Library of Tibetan Works and Archives in Dharamsala involving Doctors Yeshi Donden, Lobsang Rapgay, Pema Dorje, and Bhagwan Dash together with the Director, Mr Gyatso Tshering, is invaluable.

2. To process, correlate and synthesize such information and data already translated into a readily available clinically applicable form for the use, guidance and training of 'holistic' medicine practitioners particularly in the West – adapted and modified to modern conditions without changing its essential nature and traditional basis.

Numbers 1(b) and (c) connote first of all the predominantly academic task involving Tibetologists who are principally interested in and concerned with every aspect of Tibetan culture including Buddhism, of which medicine is only one part. These activities come principally within the purview of universities and academic research foundations which are not directly, if at all, involved with clinical medicine. There are two notable exceptions as far as I am aware personally: Dr Elisabeth Finckh, MD, in Hamburg and Dr Bhagwan Dash in Delhi.

We can do no better than follow the advice of His Holiness The Dalai Lama. Tibetan medicine can never be practised again within the context of 'the old social system' in Tibet, which 'will never be resurrected'. But, as he also says – 'The teachings of the Buddha ... [and in this case Tibetan Medicine etc.]. . . These we must preserve and promote'. The way ahead is thereby clearly indicated:

(a) Keep as intact as possible (as part of the general task of preserving the cultural heritage of Tibet) the tradition and practice of Tibetan medicine in its purest and classical form, as is already being done with great devotion in the several Tibetan Medical Centres in India and Nepal; and
(b) Adapt, without changing the fundamental basis, its theory and practice in terms of medicine and particularly holistic medicine in the West.

This is what this book is all about, an attempt to 'bridge the gap' between East and West, and above all, in medical thinking. If it ultimately serves a useful purpose to that end, then it will have been worth writing. Time alone will tell.

> We shall not cease from exploration
> And the end of all our exploring
> Will be to arrive where we started
> And know the place for the first time
> (T.S. ELIOT, *Little Gidding*)

SARVA MANGALAM

Appendix 1   Technical data for health professionals

A Guide to Tibetan Medical Urinalysis (Introduction, Methods, Materials and Results)

(Article first published in *Myrobalan* No. 3 – 'Journal of Tibetan Medicine' No. 3, published by The Study Group for Tibetan Medicine, Yalding, UK, November 1985, by Dr Lobsang Rapgay, PhD Tibetan Medicine)   Dharamsala, 29 August 1984.

Tibetan medical tradition is probably the least known system of medicine and the only documented science that enjoys an unbroken continuity of over 2500 years. Originally, Ayurveda, the Indian system of medicine was practised in Tibet, and Indian and Tibetan physicians travelled frequently between their two countries to promote and exchange medical information. However, from the seventh century, Greek, Persian and Chinese physicians visited Tibet at the invitation of Tibetan kings to share and teach their medical science. Many of the principles and clinical practices of these systems were consequently integrated into the practice of medicine by Tibetan physicians. Eventually, in the eighth century, Yuthok Yonten Gonpo, the most well known Tibetan physician in medical history, founded the present Tibetan system.

A Tibetan physician uses a number of diagnostic procedures, among which urinalysis is one of the most important. Diagnosis by urine originated from the Greeks, and this view is supported by a number of medical history texts, including the authoritative one by Desi Sangye Gyatso, a minister to the Great Fifth Dalai Lama and a medical historian and writer. He in turn quotes ancient texts and, in one such text, the Manjushri Sutra states: 'The Chinese have specialised in the art of acupuncture, the Indians in herbology, while the Greeks have perfected the methods of diagnosis (urinalysis)'.

Urinalysis is used by a Tibetan physician both for detecting a state of health, and deviation from that state. It is routinely used with other procedures not only to obtain valuable clinical information about the health of the patient but also to diagnose organic pathology, their severity and prognosis, by means and techniques entirely different from modern systems of urinalysis.

Basic Urinalysis

Urinalysis is routine for every patient seen in the physician's office, and is repeated during each visit – often daily examination may be necessary for periods ranging from one to two weeks in serious and specific diseases. When the physician is not able to examine the patient personally, examining a urine specimen is the only reliable procedure available to him. The question of whether treatment can be indicated simply on the basis of urinalysis is a matter of opinion among Tibetan physicians. However, many experienced physicians can make a complete diagnosis and decide on the treatment by just examining the urine, provided the medical history is available.

Routine urinalysis involves four basic procedures:

1. Physical examination
   a) colour
   b) odour
   c) cloudiness or steam
2. Deposits
   a) sediments
   b) cream
3. Examination of urine after change
   a) time when change occurs
   b) way change occurs
   c) post-change characteristics
4. Tests for determining diagnostic and therapeutic procedures

a) tests to determine line of treatment
b) tests to determine poisoning.

Compliances

The concentration of urine, its physical appearance and colour varies throughout a twenty-four hour period depending partly on the patient's dietary intake and partly on his activities. For instance, drinking strong tea, taking light green vegetables, intense anxiety and depression affects urine to give it a rLung characteristic. Bad-kan deposits such as glucosuria, for instance, appear often after meals, and mKhrispa deposits such as proteinuria may occur following intense physical activity.

rLung	=	Lung	=	Wind and Activity Humour
Bad-kan	=	Peh-ken	=	Phlegm and Structure Humour
mKhrispa	=	Tri-pa	=	Bile and Energy Humour

Depending on fluid intake, substances normally retained by or excreted in small amounts may appear in urine in large quantities and substances normally excreted may be retained. The temperature and climate also affect the amount of urine voided and profuse sweating reduces the amount of urine. Ingestion of diuretic medicines, certain diuretic drinks like coffee, tea and alcohol, chilling of the body, nervousness and anxiety and intravenous fluid results in an increased excretion of urine. Output of urine is significantly reduced wth decreased intake of fluid, increased intake of salts and sour food.

In order to prevent these factors from influencing the appearance and composition of urine, a set of compliances is recommended to be observed at least for a day before the examination. The main compliances are:

1) Avoid low protein diet, strong tea and light green vegetables
2) Avoid excessively rich diet, particularly spicy or oily food
3) Avoid excessive simple carbohydrates such as sugar
4) Avoid excessive fluid intake
5) Avoid sexual intercourse
6) Sleep regularly

7) Avoid strenuous physical activities
8) Avoid anxiety and depression as far as possible.

In order to observe the compliances that may be particularly relevant in the case of a patient, he should seek the physician's guidance.

Collection of Urine

In order for urinalysis to produce results, the urine must be properly collected. The first stream should be discarded since it is likely to contain contaminated bacteria and metabolic end-products. The mid-stream of the urine should be collected to fill over half a tea cup. Improper collection may invalidate the findings of the examination, particularly if the container is not clean.

Containers

Containers used for collecting urine are specified and must be thoroughly cleaned and dried before specimens are collected. Without these initial safeguards, the results will be less meaningful, if not meaningless.

Ceramic, china and even polished or brush steel containers are appropriate. Any other container, such as those made of clay, copper or iron should not be used. The colour of the container should be white, since other colours will reflect themselves in the urine.

Stirring Stick

Traditionally, three sticks from the end of a broom stick, about the length of a foot, is used. A thread is tied firmly at about an inch from one end. The other end is parted to form a triangle so that the urine may be stirred vigorously. Any wooden stick prepared in a similar way may be perfectly suitable.

Time of Urine Collection

In general, the first voided morning urine, which is the most concentrated, is the most suitable urine for analysis. Often, however, it may not be possible to obtain the first morning specimen, and in such cases a specimen voided just before breakfast may be examined.

The first morning urine should be the first specimen after 4 a.m. since any specimen collected earlier is likely to contain renal and metabolic excretions in greater proportions to the total volume of urine.

Time for Examination

The urine should be examined as early as possible, preferably at about sunrise. Examination must be done in daylight and not in electric light, since the colour of urine may not be observed clearly.

Procedure of Analysis

Unlike modern methods of urinalysis, Tibetan physicians study various physical qualities such as colour, odour and so on for pathological information about most diseases. There are nine major characteristics of urine which are studied in terms of the three stages of urine's temperature. The first four characteristics, namely colour, odour, cloudiness, and bubbles are analysed during the first stage when urine is fresh. When the urine is lukewarm, sediments and cream are analysed and finally, in the last stage when the urine is cold, the time when change occurs, the way change occurs and post-change characteristics of urine are examined.

1. Physical Examination

Involves examination of colour, odour, cloudiness (steam), and bubbles when urine is fresh. The various characteristics of each of these in pathology are categorized to form a highly effective system of reference and diagnosis.

(a) Colour

The colour is the most visible physical quality of urine. It is primarily determined by the concentration, food pigments, blood and the presence of disease. The amount of fluid intake also affects the colour. The colours during the seasons, particularly summer and winter, are distinctly affected by the presence of heat in summer and absence of it in winter.

Normally, the colour of urine is yellow or amber, primarily due to the presence of a yellow pigment, urochrome (a type of mKhrispa). During pathogenecity, the colour of urine often changes markedly due to the presence of pigments not normally present. Bile pigments may produce a yellow to yellowish-brown colour and melanin causes urine to turn into a brownish-black colour.

Colour is normally diagnostically conclusive when it corresponds to the concentration of urine. A freshly voided urine is usually transparent, but sometimes may have a turbid appearance due to the presence of phosphates and carbonates if the specimen is alkaline.

Pathologically, a reddish yellow colour urine which is concentrated means hot or inflammatory disease, while a transparent, dilute, watery urine indicates cold or non-inflammatory disease. In cases where the urine is not concentrated, then, even if it is yellowish or reddish, an inflammatory condition is not necessarily indicated. Similarly, if urine is concentrated, its dilute and watery characteristic may not indicate a non-inflammatory condition.

Since agents like dyes, vitamins, and even food affect the colour of urine, the colour may often be misleading. It is therefore of utmost importance to study the colour for pathology in terms of the other pathological characteristics of urine.

(b) Odour

The odour of urine is basically affected by metabolic end-products of food. The urine of a diabetic may have a fruity odour due to the presence of acetone (a type of bad-kan). In the case of urinary tract infection, odour may be foul smelling due to infective agents. Certain foods may impart a characteristic odour and normally, in such a case, indigestion is the cause.

Strong, pungent and concentrated urine indicates hot or inflammatory disease, while absence or minimal presence of odour means non-inflammatory disease.

(c) Cloudiness

Steam is not visible when urine is fresh and, therefore, a cold specimen of urine should be heated for a minute or so to its normal temperature in order to study its steam content. The quality of steam and rate of its disappearance are the chief factors to observe. A profuse quantity of steam which disappears rapidly indicates inflammatory disease, while a minimal steam or absence of steam means a non-inflammatory disease. A moderate quantity which disappears steadily means the presence of both hot and cold factors.

(d) Bubbles

The manner in which bubbles form, their rate and way of disappearance, colour and location are factors to be observed for pathology. In certain diseases, no bubbles form, even when urine is stirred vigorously and often this indicates severity of the disease. Very often, when it is difficult to determine the colour by looking at the urine, stir the urine and study the colour of bubbles at the rim of the container.

Bubbles of inflammatory disease are small (size of a head of a pin), forming one or two layers over the surface, and disappear rapidly after stirring. In the case of non-inflammatory disease, the bubbles are large sized or small, congested, then increase in quantity and stay for a long period of time after stirring. Bubbles are the most consistent and reliable clinical feature of urine and, therefore, should be studied in great detail.

2. Deposit Analysis

(a) Sediments

Metabolic substances normally retained, or excreted in small amounts, may appear in urine in large quantities, and substances normally excreted may be retained.

Tibetan physicians have classified sediments according to the three physiological processes of the body.

rLung sediments are like strands of hair scattered in moderate quantity in the urine, while mKhrispa sediments have a murky and cloudy appearance and generally concentrate in the centre of the urine, and bad-kan sediments, which are like sand particles, are concentrated mainly in the bottom of the container.

The quantity of sediments, and the site in which they are located, their colour and form, indicate specific pathology. Generally, profuse presence of sediments indicates inflammatory disease. However, mere presence of sediments should not necessarily mean inflammatory disease. Rather, the form and type of sediment determine the nature of pathology. If sand granules are present then either a non-inflammatory disease at a primary level is indicated or a secondary inflammatory disease.

(b) Cream

Cream is an oily formation like the greasy stain on the surface of milk. Profuse presence of cream indicates inflammatory disease while minimal or absence means non-inflammatory disease. Their location, colour, and quantity are to be observed for diagnostic purposes.

3. Examination of Urine after Change

After a minute or so, fresh voided urine turns cold, and changes in its colour and concentration take place. The time when change takes place is pathologically significant and is determined in terms of when the urine cools. Equally important for diagnostic purposes is the way in which urine changes mainly from the centre to the periphery or from the bottom to the surface of urine.

(a) Time when Change Occurs

As stated, the time when urine colour and concentration changes is pathologically significant. When change of colour and concentration occurs before urine turns cold, an inflammatory pathology is indicated. When change occurs simultaneously with the cooling of urine, generally both inflammatory and non-inflammatory conditions exist. Existence of both together does not necessarily mean that an organ is both pathologically hot or cold. Rather it means that a constitutionally non-inflammatory organ such as the kidney is affected by an inflammatory disease like infection. In order to study this procedure, the urine should be first heated to its normal temperature.

Seasonal variations, however, influence the speed and way urine changes. For instance, during winter, urine changes its colour and concentration instantly after urine has been voided, due to low temperature. While in summer, change occurs after considerable period of time after urine has been voided, due to the presence of heat.

(b) Way Change Occurs

In the case of inflammatory disease, change of colour and concentration takes place from the bottom to the surface of container, while in the case of non-inflammatory disease change occurs from the periphery to the centre of the container.

(c) Post-change Qualities

Since normally a urine specimen is available only after it has cooled, most clinical examination of urine is made in terms of the post-change characteristics, i.e. colour, bubbles, and deposits.

Each of the nine characteristics of urine is highly significant. Not only do they determine specific disease, they also determine their acuteness or chronicity and further assist to decide the type of treatment to be given. The latter data is vitally important because for each disease, a whole range of medication is available. In order to prescribe the correct combination of medicines, the physician must be aware of the severity, the pathophysiological process which is primarily involved, and the presence of secondary complications. Urine analysis provides conclusive information about these factors.

However, diagnostic accuracy comes chiefly from skill and experience, and the ability of the physician to clinically relate his findings from all the diagnostic procedures, with complete history of the patient. Because urine is so variable and easily influenced by factors that may have nothing to do with the immediate disease, urine characteristics are often deceptive. Consequently, colour of urine may often have nothing to do with the present problem of the patient.

For example, seasonal influences in summer may cause a non-inflammatory disease urine to have a yellowish colour. In the case of a chronic disease like gastric cancer, the symptoms and characteristics of urine are often suppressed by more immediate conditions of the patient. Because the patient is undergoing enormous stress and strain and is not able to cope with his condition, his urine will clearly be dominated by symptoms of his present psychological state. The bubbles will be large, and disappear rapidly, and consequently a physician who fails to take a complete medical history will make an incorrect diagnosis and miss the real problem of the person.

The guideline for beginners is to observe as many conformities as possible in the characteristics of urine. For instance, if the colour does not agree by findings of concentration, bubbles and deposits supporting each other, diagnosis should be made on the basis of conformity of these major characteristics. Initially, when training to examine urine, analysing it in terms of the three pathophysiological processes is absolutely essential. The first of the three, rLung (activity humour) is associated with the function of the central and secondary nervous systems while mKhrispa (energy humour) is related to the activities of the endocrine and secretory systems. Bad-kan (structure humour), the last of the three, is associated with the digestive and fluid systems of the body. Each of these three is physiologically identified with specific organs, tissues, and mechanisms of the body, and therefore, being able to determine their involvement and pathogenecity in the disease process, provides essential data for arriving at a correct diagnosis. For instance, take a urine which is transparent, watery in colour, with large sized bubbles that are sparse in quantity and disappear instantly after stirring. The size of bubbles, transparency and colour indicate rLung pathology. However, the sparse quantity of bubbles and their rapid and erratic disappearances clearly means the presence of an inflammatory condition.

Clinically, there are two sites that are normally associated with such urine characteristics. They are the stomach and kidneys. The stomach, as the site of pathology in this case, is instantly ruled out because both the dilute and watery nature of urine as well as sparse quantity of bubbles clearly indicate a kidney organ involvement. This is because, though both the organs are intrinsically bad-kan sites, the kidney is predominantly a fluid bad-kan organ while the stomach is a solid (earth) bad-kan organ. The final diagnosis therefore, is inflammation of kidneys.

Normal Healthy Urine

Colour:	amber or straw
Odour:	moderate and tolerable
Cloudiness:	moderate
Bubbles:	moderate sized (about the size of small peas), moderate in quantity (spread evenly over surface of urine in not more than two layers), do not disappear instantly nor do they stand completely after stirring.
Sediments:	moderate, cover the surface
Cream:	moderate

Time when change occurs: about the same time when urine turns cold

Way change occurs: from the peripheral to the centre

Post-change characteristics: clear, straw or amber coloured, with moderate amount of sediments.

Clinically, a healthy urine with all the characteristics mentioned is rarely encountered.

Pathological Urine

Since Tibetan clinical medicine is presented in terms of the three pathophysiological processes, urine characteristics are also similarly classified.

rLung Urine

Colour:	bluish, water and transparent
Odour:	Faint or none
Cloudiness:	moderate and not significant
Bubbles:	large sized as big as 'the eyes of a buffalo', stand for some time after stirring, and disappear amidst moderate sized bubbles which may stand for a longer period depending on pathology
Sediments:	generally none; however, in certain rLung diseases, hair-like strands of deposit are present
Cream:	none

In determining rLung disease, though all the clinical features of urine are important, the colour and bubble structures are the most conclusive. Though rLung bubbles are described as large sized, it does not mean that all the bubbles will be large sized. Rather, most of the bubbles are moderate sized (size of peas) and, on stirring, a few large sized bubbles appear amid these moderate sized bubbles. When urine is bluish, clear, and large bubbles appear on stirring which disappear instantly when stirring ceases, a secondary condition of inflammation is indicated. This is diagnosed as inflammatory rLung. However, when urine is clear and the bubbles stand after stirring, it is non-inflammatory rLung.

Though inflammatory rLung diseases may sometimes contain a profuse quantity of bubbles, the bubbles are more transparent than in the case of non-inflammatory rLung disease, and disappear in an erratic fashion. In non-inflammatory rLung the bubbles are dense, making it difficult to see the bottom of the container clearly, and when an attempt is made to clear the bubbles at the centre of the container with the stick, the bubbles continue to stand.

Often colour of rLung urine may not be bluish – it may be light yellowish or slightly tainted red, except in summer, when the heat influences primary rLung urine to acquire such a colour: during other seasons, it generally means the presence of an inflammatory secondary condition.

mKhrispa Urine

Colour: reddish yellow, chocolate or oil-like
Odour: strong and pungent
Cloudiness: profuse and persists for a short period
Bubbles: small sized (about the size of a pin-head), not congested like bad-kan bubbles (do not increase into many layers like bad-kan on stirring), and disappear instantly
Sediments: profuse and concentrated in the surface, middle and bottom of container depending on location of disease; the sediments are murky and cloudy
Cream: profuse and mainly concentrated in the centre
Time change occurs: before urine turns cold
Way change occurs: from bottom to the surface of the container
Post-change characteristics: cloudy and concentrated, and reddish yellow, small sized bubbles.

Cloudiness, concentration and bubbles are clinically the most significant features in mKhrispa urine diagnosis. The colour is often deceptive and can only have clinical value if urine is concentrated. Generally the way to measure concentration of urine is by observing how clearly the bottom of the container can be seen. If it is seen as clearly as in the case of water, the urine is dilute and means a non-inflammatory disease. On the other hand, if it is murky, the bottom may not be seen, indicating an inflammatory disease.

Often colour of urine which is yellowish or reddish may be deceptive. In order to determine colour, tilt the container slightly and observe the rim of the tilted side. If it is clear, consider a non-inflammatory disease.

Normally, bubbles of mKhrispa or inflammatory disease are

small (size of a pin's head), congested but not profuse, and do not form more than a few layers on stirring, unlike in the case of bad-kan disease. The urine is concentrated and the bubbles disappear rapidly even while stirring. After a minute or even less, the centre of the container becomes clear of bubbles and finally only a few may be observed at the edge of urine.

Bad-kan Urine

Colour: white like milk but generally water

Odour: minimal or none

Cloudiness: minimal and disappears before change takes place

Bubbles: congested, small sized, increase profusely on stirring, and stand for considerable amount of time after stirring; in fact rarely do bubbles disappear at all

Sediments: minimal or none but, in metabolic and kidney bad-kan diseases, sand granules are present at bottom of container

Cream: none

Time change occurs: after urine has turned cold

Way change occurs: from periphery to centre of container

Post-change characteristics: white, generally clear, congested and profuse bubbles which stand.

The bubble is the chief clinical feature to observe in bad-kan urine. Congested bubbles, which are small sized and increase on stirring profusely clearly indicate bad-kan disease.

However, colour often determines location of disease, for instance, a urine with bad-kan bubbles that stands but has a yellowish brown colour. The colour is clinically associated with abdominal diseases particularly that of the stomach and duodenum. Since the stomach is associated with bad-kan it may be inferred from the urine that a bad-kan pathology of the stomach is present. The yellowish colour may indicate the presence of inflammation also.

Kidneys are another major bad-kan organ but, since it is primarily associated with fluid, the bubbles are not profuse, nor do they stand for very long. Moreover, the urine is watery and dilute in most cases.

mKhrispa–rLung Urine
Colour: yellowish light and clear
Odour: moderate and slightly pungent
Cloudiness: moderate quantity and duration
Bubbles: small to moderate sized with sporadic large sized,
               which instantly disappear after stirring
Sediments: slightly concentrated but generally clear
Cream: minimal

The differential diagnosis for this kind of urine is, notably, sinusitis, flu, hay fever, and enteritis. However, there are certain distinctions in each case. In the case of sinusitis and hay fever, the colour and concentration are clearer than in the case of common cold or flu. In the case when cough is present, the bubbles are profuse and moderate in size and form loose layers on stirring. In the case of enteritis, the urine is not concentrated but more yellowish with sporadic rLung sized bubbles that disappear instantly.

Bad-kan – rLung Urine
Colour: watery and clear
Odour: none or minimal
Cloudiness: minimal and disappears before change occurs
Bubbles: small sized, congested bubbles with sporadic
               large sized bubbles that appear on stirring and
               stand for some time after stirring
Sediments: generally minimal except in cases of indigestion
Cream: none

Bad-kan – mKhrispa Urine
Colour: reddish yellow, dark like oil or chocolate
Odour: pungent and strong
Cloudiness: profuse but moderate duration
Bubbles: small to moderate sized that stand after stirring
Sediments: murky, or granules may be present
Cream: moderate

This kind of urine is typical in the case of diseases with jaundice as a major symptom. However, in the case of gall stone, the urine is clearer with fewer bubbles that disappear erratically on stirring.

Complex Bad-kan Disease

Colour:	yellowish brown and concentrated
Odour:	strong and pungent
Cloudiness:	moderate to profuse depending on presence of fever
Bubbles:	small to moderate sized, congested, that stand for some time after stirring
Sediments:	moderate and concentrated mainly in the centre: rim of container may appear clear
Cream:	moderate in cases of inflammatory complex bad-kan disease

Complex bad-kan disease is a pathological state involving all the three pathophysiological processes primarily in the abdominal region. There are three main stages of disease namely, first or inflammatory, second and third or non-inflammatory. They correspond to severe gastritis, ulcer, and perforated ulcer. Urine will be distinct for each stage. In the first stage, it will be yellowish and inflammatory in character, while in the second it will have both inflammatory and non-inflammatory characteristics. During the third stage, urine will contain blood cells and small sized bubbles that stand.

Common Cold or Flu Urine

Colour:	light yellowish and concentrated in centre
Odour:	pungent if fever present
Bubbles:	diffuse, and covers surface in a layer to two but not profuse, moderate sized that disappear erratically with a hissing sound

Common cold urine may be easily mistaken for a variety of other diseases such as enteritis and hay fever. The chief feature of common cold urine is the slightly murky and concentrated sediments in the centre, while the rim is clear. In the case of enteritis and hay fever, the urine is clear and more yellowish.

Meningitis

Colour:	yellowish red, slightly concentrated
Odour:	strong and pungent

Cloudiness: profuse
Bubbles: small, diffuse but do not increase much on stirring, and disappear rapidly
Sediments: moderate
Cream: minimal or none

A point to note is that, in most cases of inflammatory disease of the nervous system, the urine tends to have a reddish colour.

Intestinal Colic
Colour: yellow and clear
Odour: moderate
Bubbles: small to moderate, may be sparse and disappear rapidly
Sediments: minimal or none

In most cases of organic inflammatory disease, presence of fever will affect the concentration, cloudiness and odour of urine distinctly. When fever is present, urine will be more concentrated, darker in colour, with a pungent odour. In case fever is absent, urine will be transparent, particularly if inflammation is present in a cold constitutional organ.

Weak Digestive Syndrome
Colour: whitish and concentrated
Odour: moderate, often odour of indigested food
Bubbles: small, congested with occasional rLung bubbles that stand
Sediments: metabolic end-products may be present, often giving urine a milky turbid appearance

Dyspepsia
Colour: reddish yellow or milk white
Odour: food
Bubbles: small, diffused and stand for a while after stirring

Generally, dyspepsia caused by eating unwholesome food or overeating greasy and spicy food, if left untreated, affects the whole metabolic function. The digestive heat is impaired, resulting in a permanent weak digestive system. Consequently, further disregard of dietary habits will cause severe inflammatory conditions or atrophy of bad-kan (mucus) causing tumoural growths in the abdominal region.

Flatulence
Colour: water and dilute
Odour: minimal
Bubbles   large sized among profuse moderate sized bubbles that may stand for a while
Sediments: none visible though some may be noticed when inflammatory conditions are present

Enteritis
Colour: reddish yellow and basically clear
Odour: pungent
Bubbles: small, with occasional large sized bubbles, sparse in quantity, may sometimes cover the surface, disappear rapidly
Sediments: generally none, but sometimes granules may be present

Hepatitis
Colour: oil like or chocolate
Odour: pungent and strong
Cloudiness: profuse but persists for a long time
Bubbles: yellowish colour, small to moderate sized, congested and stand for a long time
Sediments: concentrated and murky
Cream: moderate

Acute Cholecystitis
Colour: yellowish and concentrated
Odour: pungent
Cloudiness: profuse but does not persist
Bubbles: small, yellowish but not profuse (on stirring layer or two may form) and disappear rapidly, though

small sized bubbles may stand round the rim of
urine.

Cholelithiasis

Colour:	yellowish but transparent
Odour:	moderate
Bubbles:	small to few moderate sized, sparse in quantity and disappear erratically with a hissing sound
Sediments:	generally clear but may be slightly concentrated sometimes
Cream:	circumscribed, and size of a frog's egg are found scattered over surface

When pain is a prominent, clinical symptom in the case of any
disease, the bubbles generally are sparse to moderate in quantity,
often large size and disappear erratically with a hissing sound.

Intestinal Worms

Colour:	whitish yellow and transparent
Bubbles:	sparse with a few large sized that disappear entirely after stirring

Pneumonia

Colour:	reddish yellow and slightly concentrated
Odour:	moderate
Cloudiness:	moderate and persistent
Bubbles:	small to moderate sized, slightly profuse but transparent to see the bottom of container (in abdominal diseases, bubbles are equal or more in quantity but are dense and prevent seeing the bottom of container) and disappear rapidly
Sediments:	slightly concentrated or murky; may be transparent

In respiratory diseases, urine generally appears yellowish red and,
when cough is a major symptom, layers of bubbles form but are
loose and sit on top of each other. Generally the sizes of such
bubbles are moderate but may be slightly larger; they generally
tend to disappear with a hissing sound.

Bronchitis

Colour: yellowish white and transparent

Odour: moderate

Bubbles: small to moderate sized, congested but not profuse and disappear gradually

Asthma

Colour: whitish and clear

Odour: moderate sized with few interspersing large sized bubbles, profuse in quantity and stand for a while

Functional Heart Disease

Colour: light reddish or bluish; transparent

Bubbles: large sized that do not stand for long, moderate quantity

In organic heart diseases, colour of urine is yellowish red, concentrated, and bubbles are profuse and smaller in size.

Rheumatic Heart Disease

Colour: yellowish and slightly concentrated

Odour: moderate

Bubbles: large sized, interspersed with moderate size bubbles which disappear gradually

Hypertension urine characteristics vary. In the case of rLung hypertension, urine is generally transparent, bluish and has a moderate quantity of bubbles. In the case of organic hypertension, such as in coronary heart disease, urine is concentrated, yellowish red, and bubbles are smaller in size with occasional large sized ones.

Anaemia

Colour: bluish clear and slightly tainted yellow in inflammatory cases

Bubbles: various sized, congested and profuse that stand

When fever is present, urine is slightly yellowish and the bubbles may be less profuse and tend to disappear after stirring. However, when no fever is present, urine is bluish, watery and huge quantities of bubbles form and increase doubly on stirring, filling the whole container.

Tumorous growth

Colour: Yellowish light or dark reddish brown

Odour: pungent or moderate

Bubbles: small to moderate, slightly congested and stand. In cases of benign tumour and non-inflammatory cancer, bubbles are sparse and disappear erratically

Sediments: concentrated in centre; on tapping surface of urine with stirring stick, small oily shooting bubbles form

Cream: circumscribed and size of frog's eggs spread all over surface

Generally, tumorous growths are classified as either inflammatory or non-inflammatory. Non-inflammatory tumours are benign, while inflammatory tumours mean malignancy. However, site of growth will also determine the nature of tumour. For instance, if a benign tumour occurs in a constitutionally hot organ, urine will be characterised by both hot and cold clinical features.

Arthritis

Colour: yellowish red or brown and generally transparent

Odour: moderate, may be strong sometimes

Bubbles: small to moderate sized, not profuse in quantity but cover surface of urine when stirred and disappear rapidly

When tenderness and pain are the chief symptoms, bubbles tend to be moderate to large sized, sparse and disappear erratically with a hissing sound. In case of swelling, urine is clearer and bubbles stand for a longer time.

Major Differential Diagnoses

Clinical features of urine may be easily mistaken for a number of diseases. Only clinical skill and experience can determine their differences. Some of the important differential diagnoses have been mentioned already. Tibetan medical texts discuss six main diseases whose clinical features may be mistaken for each other, and they are discussed here.

1. Colour

Reddish colour of urine in the case of rLung fever and general fever (without rLung) can cause the physician to take one for the other. However, careful observation will help to make the distinction. rLung fever will, apart from fever features, contain rLung characteristics, namely it will be clear with large bubbles. In the case of general fever, however, urine will be concentrated, even murky, with small bubbles that disappear rapidly.

2. Transparency and Sediments

Light, whitish coloured urine with sediment, may be easily mistaken for a non-inflammatory disease. However, presence of sediment is clinically more significant and consequently diagnosis should be based on its presence. The light, whitish colour of urine is secondary. Similarly, if sediment is not present in urine which is yellowish red in colour, the colour is insignificant and the diagnosis should be based on the absence of sediment.

3. Colour and Bubbles

The watery, bluish colour of urine in the case of hidden fever (fever of a constitutionally cold organ, or fever occurring during winter), low blood pressure and cold kidney diseases may easily be mistaken for one another. However, their distinguishing clinical features are clear on careful observation. In the case of hidden fever, bubbles which are small and disappear clearly indicate the element of fever. On the other hand, in the case of low blood pressure, bubbles are large rLung sized and stand a while.

Factors to Keep in Mind During Urinalysis

Many of the causes that determine colour and composition of urine both during health and pathology have been discussed at earlier stages. However, there are certain points to be kept in mind during urine examination.

Humoural Constitutional Predisposition

There are seven humoural constitutions, chief of which are the three humoural processes namely rLung, mKhrispa and bad-kan. Normally constitutional body is determined by pulse examination and questioning when a person is physically healthy. That is why, during medical history taking, it is recommended that the patient is asked about his constitutional humour. In case he is not able to provide one, questioning him about his normal diet, activity and predisposition may give an idea of his constitutional humour.

Seasonal Factor

Seasons play a vital role in determining urine features. It is recommended that the physician keeps in mind the season during which he is examining the urine, particularly if it happens to be winter or summer. Generally, summer pathological urine will acquire inflammatory characteristics. Keeping in mind the seasonal and other factors such as drugs, diet, activity and so on and their influence on urine features, so the urine should be examined. Clinical features discovered in urine should be compared against clinical information in medical texts before deciding on a diagnosis.

However, making a complete diagnosis on the basis of urinalysis alone is not suggested. If nothing else, history should be taken carefully before examining urine.

4. Tests to Determine Diagnostic and Therapeutic Procedures

When the physician has time, and the case is serious, requiring utmost caution in treatment, additional tests may be carried out.

(a) Tests for Determining Line of Treatment

The most common and effective test to determine line of treatment is carried out by heating urine to its normal temperature if the specimen is cold. A powder of the drug which is to be tested is sprinkled on the surface of urine. Sprinkle on one side of the surface in order to leave space for testing other medicines.

If the powder spreads gradually over the whole surface of urine as soon as it is sprinkled, the particular drug is very suitable for the patient. If the powder spreads instantly and in a rapid fashion, though the drug is suitable and may be recommended, it is less effective than another drug which may spread gradually over the surface. In case the powder sinks gradually to the bottom without any major spreading, the drug is not suitable and should not be used. If the powder sinks rapidly, the drug is again not suitable and should not be used. In conducting such tests, it is suggested that drugs should not be randomly tested. Rather only those drugs which are normally indicated for the disease and which may be causing doubts in the physician's mind as to which particular one is to be indicated at this stage, should be tested for good results.

(b) Tests for Determining Diagnosis

Though there are a number of tests for determining the diagnosis, here only those tests to determine poisoning are mentioned.

In case poisoning is suspected, the physician should spit his fresh saliva into the urine of the patient. If the saliva floats on the surface, poisoning is not present. If saliva sinks to the bottom instantly, poisoning is present.

Another test is by taking a strand of hair from any person other than the patient. Cast it into urine. If it coils and has a burnt appearance, poisoning is indicated. Otherwise, it means no poisoning.

Conclusion

No amount of literature or urinalysis can substitute for the importance of studying the technique under a competent physician.

While basic procedures of how to diagnose disease are provided here, many subtle aspects of urine examination have been deliberately left out to prevent confusion to the beginner for whom this work is intended. Additional information based on personal observations in the clinic, and which is not available elsewhere, has been added to provide the beginner with a clearer guideline to work upon.

Appendix 2   General Information

1. Tibetan Medical Texts and Commentaries

It is said that Dr Yeshi Donden has a private library of over 400 Tibetan Medical Texts and Commentaries, and there are more. The following is just a modest selection of some of the notable ones:

Bai Dur Snon Po (4 Volumes)
Being the text of 'Gso ba rig pa'i bstan bcos sman bla'i dgons rgyan rgyud bzi'i gsal byed bai dur snon po'i ma llika'
Sde-srid Sangs-rgyas-rGya-mtsho's detailed synthetic treatise on the Rgyud bzi, the fundamental exposition of Tibetan ayurvedic medicine
Reproduced from a print the 1888-1892 blocks preserved in the Lha-sa lcags-po-ri rig-byed-'gro-phan-glin
by
T.Y. Tashigangpa
Volumes I, II, III & IV
Rtsa rgyud dan bsad rgyud
Leh
1973

Techniques of Lamaist Medical Practice
Being the text of
Man ngag yon tan rgyud kyi lhan thabs zug rngu'i tsha gdung sel ba'i katpu ra dus min 'chi zhags gcod pa'i ral gri
by
Sde-srid Sangs-rgyas-rGya-mtsho

Reproduced from a print from the 1952 blocks edited by
the Venerable Mkhyen-rab-nor-bu
Leh
1970

Gso rig bstan bcos mtha' dag gi snin po rnams phyogs gcig tu
bsdus pa man nag rin chen 'byun gnas
A treatise on Tibetan ayurvedic practice containing numerous
instructions and medical formulae
by
'Jam-dpal-rdo-rje
Reproduced from a print from blocks carved through the efforts of
Dpal-'byor (the Dem-chi of the Lha-khan Ser-po of Dolonor) from
the library of Prof. Dr Lokesh Chandra
Leh
1975

Gso rig gdos pa kun 'byung (3 Volumes)
An exhaustive treatise on Tibetan medicine
by
Gong-sman Dkon-mchog-bde-legs
Photographically reproduced from the Sman-sgom
Bsam-pa-don-grub manuscript from Ladakh
with an English introduction by
Lharje Tashi Yangphel Tashigang
Volume(s) I (II & III)
Leh
1971

Man nag lhan thabs kyi lde mig
Explanation of difficult terms occurring in the Sde-srid's 'Man nag
lhan thabs'
by
Nag-dban-dpal-bzan-po
Zin rig mdzes rgyan bdud rtsi sman mdzod
A medical formulary based on Kon-sprul's 'Zin tig gces btus bdud
rtsi'i thigs pa'
by
O-rgyan-bstan-'dzin

Gces bsdus 'Chi med nor bui' phren ba
A medical formulary
by
Dbon-sprul Karma-ratna
Reproduced from rare xylographic prints and tracings
Leh
1973

Gso spyad sno sbyor tshogs kyi man nag rin chen 'khruns dpe
bstan
A Tibetan botanical treatise on the recognition of medicinal plants
reproduced from a rare incomplete manuscript from Khams by
Tondup Tashi
Leh
1974

Slob ma la phan p a'i zin tig
A collection of instructions on Tibetan medicine and treatment
by
Gtsan-sman Dar-ma-mgon-po
Volumes I & II

Bye ba rin bsrel (2 Volumes)
A reproduction of the 18th century Sde-dge redaction of a version
of the collected instructions on medical practice of Zur-mkhar
Mnam-nid-rdo-rje. Reproduced from a print from the library of
Pepung Ongen Rimpoche
Volumes I & II
Gangtok
1977

Fundamentals of Tibetan Medical Practice
Lha-sa Sman-rtsis-khan prints of works of Mkhyen-ran-nor-bu, 'Ju
Mi-pham, Chos-grags-rgya-mtsho, and 'Jam-mgon Kon-sprul
Smanrtsis Shesrig Spendzod
Leh
1974

The Gist Prescriptions of the Tibetan Traditional Medicines
Ngo mT'sar-'K'rul-Gyi-Me-Long.

A comprehensive list of Tibetan Medical Literature is available
from:
Dr T.W. Tashigangpa,
L-125, Laxmi Nagar,
Delhi 110092, India.

2. Training in Tibetan Medicine

(a) T.M.I., The Tibetan Medical Institute
Khara Danda Road
Dharamsala
Distt. Kangra
(H.P.) India

(b) Kopan Tibetan Medical Centre
Kathmandu
Kingdom of Nepal

3. Organizations Concerned with the Promotion of Tibetan Medicine

Dharma Therapy Trust (incorporating the Study Group for
Tibetan medicine) U.K.,
'Lower Fosse Cottage'
Oakhill
Bath, Avon, U.K.

Foundation for International Medical Exchange
16250
Grove Street
Berkeley CA 94709 U.S.A.

Kagyu Samye Ling Tibetan Centre
Eskdalemuir
Nr. Langholm
Dumfriesshire DG1 3OL
Scotland

Library of Tibetan Works & Archives
Gangchen Kyishong
Dharamsala
Distt. Kangra
H.P. India

Rigpa Meditation Centre
44 St. Paul's Crescent
London NW1 9TN
U.K.

The Society for Tibetan Medicine
107 East 31st Street
New York 10016
U.S.A.

Vajradhatu
1345 Spruce Street
Boulder CO 80302
U.S.A.

4. Subject Matter Analysis of the rGyud bZhi, the Four Medical Tantras (material which has been translated into English)

1st Tantra

(rTza-rGyud) or Root Tantra (Mula Tantra in Sanskrit). There are two translations, one by the Ven. Jhampa Kelsang with annotations by Dr Yeshi Donden, which is published by the Library of Tibetan Works and Archives as Part 1 of 'The Ambrosia Heart Tantra'. The second translation as yet unpublished has been made by Barry Clark.

2nd Tantra

(bShad rGyud) or Explanatory Tantra (Akhyata Tantra in Sanskrit). Part 2 of the 'Ambrosia Heart Tantra' mentioned above contains a translation of half of this Tantra. There is also another translation of this by Barry Clark. 'gSorig' No. 9, 1985 also contains four chapters – 'The Practice and Theory of Therapeutics in Tibetan Medicine'. Chapters I–XXXI, i.e. the whole of this Tantra have also been translated by Rechung Rinpoche – see *Tibetan Medicine*, pp. 29–92.

3rd Tantra

(Man ngag rGyud) or Oral Instruction Tantra (Upadesa-Tantra in Sanskrit). This Tantra contains 92 chapters. Very little of it has been translated, but some of the subject matter will be found in a condensed form on specific diseases, their causes, symptoms and treatment. This is published in 'gSorig' No. 2, 1981, by the Library of Tibetan Works and Archives. Terence Clifford has translated the 77th, 78th and 79th chapters on Tibetan psychiatry – see also Dr Stanley Frye who has translated Chapter 49 from the Russian, on the Treatment of Colic.

4th Tantra

(Phyi-ma rGyud), last text, or the text of the Appendices (Uttaratantra in Sanskrit). A text on 'Pulse Diagnosis' appears in 'tSorig' No. 1 (1980) by Dr Yeshi Donden which is taken from Chapter 1 of this Tantra. Chapters 1 and 2 dealing with the examination of the pulse and veins and the urine have also been translated by Rechung Rinpoche.
Dr Bhagwan Dash is at present translating the Four Medical Tantras into English and Professor Emmerick is translating them into the German language.

5. Structured Syllabus for the Further Study of Tibetan Medicine

Introduction

The study of Tibetan medicine is envisaged in the West in three stages.

1. The introductory stage or mastery of elementary principles over a period of two years which involves twenty meetings (i.e. ten per annum) plus home study. This is the only possibility at this point in the evolution of the group's activities and the following syllabus applies solely to this aspect.
2. An intermediate course of instruction under the personal tutelage of a qualified doctor of Tibetan medicine. The duration of such a course, its form and actual syllabus is yet to be determined, being totally dependent on the eventual presence of a qualified Tibetan doctor.
3. At the moment solely by enrolment for the full five year course in Dharamsala can a student fully qualify. Providing stages 1 and 2 could be fulfilled it may be that a system of credits might be possible so the actual study period in Dharamsala could be reduced. The possibility of this would be subject for future discussion with those concerned in Dharamsala and at this point in time is hypothetical.

Stage 1 The Introductory Group Study Syllabus

Based on the 'Ambrosia Heart Tantra' which is the Root Tantra or rTza-rGyud, comprising the first of the four basic treatises to tradition, plus the first half of the Explanatory Tantra.

1st Session   Introduction and enumeration of subjects
2nd Session   The basis of illness
3rd Session   Diagnosis and symptoms
4th Session   Methods of healing
5th Session   The enumeration of metaphors
6th Session   Synthesis of the explanatory tantra
7th Session   The manner of the formation of the body
8th Session   Similes for the body
9th Session   The anatomy of the body
10th Session Characteristics of the body
11th Session The actions and classifications of the body
12th Session Signs of death
13th Session The causes of illnesses

14th Session The conditions contributing to illnesses
15th Session The manner of entrance of illnesses
16th Session The characteristics of illnesses
17th Session The classification of illnesses
18th Session Continual daily behaviour
19th Session Seasonal behaviour
20th Session Occasional behaviour

General Plan of the Introductory Stage

1. Group meetings for discussion on subject material already prepared at home.
2. This activity to be supplemented with relevant material from tape-recordings of Dr Yeshi Donden's lectures already given in the UK, plus other tapes that could become available, i.e. if there were a demand. Reading of standard textbooks in the English language would also be recommended.
3. In addition, qualified Teachers, Rinpoches, Geshes, etc., or others resident in the UK or Europe and overseas correspondents could be asked to amplify specific subject material pertinent to each section by actual teaching or dissertation either given in person or by the exchange of tapes.

Standard Textbooks in the English Language

Of more recent publication, Elisabeth Finckh's *Foundations of Tibetan Medicine*, vols. I and II, based directly on translations of the rGud bZhi represents one of the finest expositions of traditional Tibetan medicine according to the Buddhist medical texts.

Terry Clifford's book *Tibetan Buddhist Medicine and Psychiatry* on the other hand whilst being an excellent general treatise emphasizes the psychiatric aspect of Tibetan medicine, which by the way is traditionally very considerable. Dr Yeshi Donden's even more recent book *Health through Balance* is excellent, comprehensive and fundamental. Professor Namkhai Norbu's excellent short work *On Birth and Life – a Treatise on Tibetan Medicine*, gives in considerable detail much essential information on dietetics.

This present volume has a different purpose, i.e. to introduce practitioners of other medicines, particularly Western, to the subject of Tibetan medicine. While providing basic information about a number of these – osteopathy, homoeopathy and herbal medicine for instance – primarily for the non-informed everywhere (including Tibetan physicians), it seeks to emphasize the common ground between all systems of medicine. The basic primer and reference book in the English language is, of course, Rechung Rinpoche's book *Tibetan Medicine*.

To summarize:
1. Basic primer and reference book – Rechung Rinpoche's book.
2. Translations of texts with commentary presented in a very traditional context – Elisabeth Finckh's two volumes.
3. Basic principles and clinical Tibetan medicine – Dr Yeshi Donden's book.
4. Tibetan medicine basics and dietetics – Professor Namkhai Norbu's book.
5. Tibetan medicine with an emphasis on psychiatry – Terry Clifford's book.
6. The present volume presenting the subject in a more general way plus acting as a bridge between other systems of medicine and the Tibetan discipline.

Already a prolific lecturer and writer of articles and monographs, Dr Lobsang Rapgay promises to soon be one of the most important sources of knowledge of Tibetan medicine in the English language.

6. Names and Addresses of Tibetan Doctors

Dr Tenzin Choedhak & Staff Physicians,
Tibetan Medical Institute,
Khara Danda Road,
Dharamsala,
Distt. Kangra,
(H.P.), India

Dr Barry Clark,
c/o Library of Tibetan Works & Archives,
Gangchen Kyishong,
Dharamsala,
Distt. Kangra,
(H.P.), India.

Dr Lobsang Dolma,
McLeod Ganj,
Dharamsala,
Distt. Kangra,
(H.P.), India.

Dr Yeshi Donden,
'Ashok Niwas',
McLeod Ganj,
Dharamsala,
Distt. Kangra,
(H.P.), India.

Dr Pema Dorjee,
Siddhartha Vihara Dispensary,
P.O. Itanagar-97111
(A.P.), India.

Dr Lobsang Rapgay, Ph.D. (Tibetan Medicine),
Tshering House,
193 McLeod Ganj,
Dharamsala,
Distt. Kangra,
(H.P.), India.

Ven. Dr Trogawa Rinpoche,
c/o Rigpa Fellowship,
P.O. Box 7326,
Santa Cruz, CA 95061
U.S.A.

7. The Tibetan Medical Institute

This was formerly known as the Tibetan Medical Centre which was inaugurated in 1961 by the 14th Dalai Lama of Tibet. During the intervening six years since the author was last in Dharamsala, the Medical Centre and School has made fantastic strides, in developing its premises, equipment and amenities, and has also expanded its activities enormously. The comparatively tiny wooden building that originally housed the Medical Centre in McLeod Ganj, not far from Thekchen Chöling, His Holiness' residence and the Temple, is still apparently retained as a Clinic, but pales now beside the new brick and concrete buildings to be found a little lower down from the Library and just above the Kotwali bazar, the beginning of lower Dharamsala.

The Tibetan Medical Institute houses a Tibetan Medical College which is currently training on a five-year full-time course some fifty students. Additionally three students are attending the associated School of Astrological Studies. Dr Pasang Yonten is Principal of the College and Professor Jampa G. Dhakton supervises the Astrology department. In addition there are the Out-Patient Clinics and a fifteen-bed hospital with a dispensary and the latter building is now the headquarters of the Institute. Dr Tenzin Choedhak assisted by Dr J. Tashi, the Dalai Lama's Senior and Junior Physicians, are in charge.

The Pharmacy is supervised by Dr Tenzin Namgyal. At present 187 different medicines are made in the traditional way with herbs, gems, metal and animal extracts, including the Jewel Pills (see Chapter 7). The pharmacy is capable of producing over 1000 different medicines, many of which are exported all over the world. Research is under the direction of Dr S. Tsering.

The Tibetan Medical and Astrological Museum was officially opened by His Holiness the Dalai Lama on 6 March 1976. It displays various raw drugs, surgical instruments, medical and astrological charts, thangkas, icons and other materials of interest. The Shrine-Room contains beautiful thangkas both of the Medicine Buddha and His Mandala, also statues of the Eight Medicine Buddhas presented by His Holiness in July 1982.

The Institute was formerly, before his untimely decease,

directed by Mr Lobsang Samden Taklha, the brother of His Holiness, assisted by his wife Mrs Namlha Samden-Taklha, who is now the Director.

The address is: Khara Danda Road,
Dharamsala,
Distt. Kangra,
(Himachal Pradesh),
India.

Notes

1 Tibetan Medical Philosophy

1. B.C. Olschak, 'The Art of Healing in Ancient Tibet' from *An Introduction to Tibetan Medicine*, The Tibetan Review, 1976, edited by Dawa Norbu.
2. Dr Bhagwan Dash, formerly Deputy Advisor (Ayurveda) Ministry of Health and Family Planning, New Delhi, *Tibetan Medicine – Yogasataka*, Library of Tibetan Works & Archives, Dharamsala.
3. Dr Elisabeth Finckh, *Foundations of Tibetan Medicine*, volume 1, Watkins, London.
4. *Fundamentals of Tibetan Medicine according to the rGyud-bzhi*, Tibetan Medical Centre, Dharamsala, 1981.
5. Dr Bhagwan Dash, *Tibetan Medicine*.
6. Yanlag brGyad-pa Chhenpo – eight great branches of medicine.
   1. General medicine
   2. Paediatrics
   3. Obstetrics
   4. Psychiatry
   5. Traumatic injuries
   6. Toxicology
   7. Geriatrics
   8. Sexology
7. Guru Padmasambhava, the great Indian Pandita who took Buddhism to Tibet and who also founded the Nyingmapa (the Old Sect) which still exists today.
8. The literature on Tibetan medicine is vast and a selection can be found in university libraries and the Wellcome Institute of the History of Medicine. A comprehensive list of Tibetan Medical Literature is available from Dr T.W. Tashigangpa, L-125, Laxmi Nagar, Delhi 110092, India.
9. Marianne Winder, 'Tibetan Medicine Compared with Ancient and Mediaeval Western Medicine', Bulletin of Tibetology, Sikkim

284

Research Institute of Tibetology, Gangtok, 1981, No. 1.

10. Dr Yeshi Donden, 'The Modernity of Tibetan Medicine' from *An Introduction to Tibetan Medicine*, The Tibetan Review, 1976, edited by Dawa Norbu.

11. S.T. Phuntsog and N.G. Namgyal, *Evolution of Tibetan Medicine*, Herbalcure, Hyderabad, 3 vols. (1–2), No. 3.

12. Dr Bhagwan Dash, *Indian Contribution to Tibetan Medicine*, The Tibetan Review, 1976.

13. Dr Bhagwan does not give the titles, but they were composed by K'ung-trul Jig-me nam-mK'ai dorje during 1937–50 and published by the Centre in 1972.

Note: For more detailed notes on the history of Tibetan Medicine, see 'Notes on the History of Tibetan Medicine' by Enrico dell Angelo, *gSORIG* no. 8, 1984, Library of Tibetan Works & Archives.

2 Buddhist Tantra, Cosmology and Symbolism Relevant to Tibetan Medicine

1. Lama Anagarika Govinda, *Foundations of Tibetan Mysticism*, Rider and Company, London, 1960.

2. Ven. Trungpa Rinpoche, *The Dawn of Tantra*, Shambala Publications Inc., Berkeley and London, 1975, résumé from pages 2 & 5.

3. Herbert V. Guenther, *The Life and Teachings of Naropa*, Oxford University Press, 1963.

4. From a verbal commentary on the Six Realms given by Francesca Fremantle.

5. Ven. Trungpa Rinpoche, 'Space Therapy', *The Middle Way*, Vol. 1, No. 3, November 1975.

6. Thinley Norbu, *The Magic Dance*, Jewel Publishing House, New York, 1985.

7. Dr Tenzin Choedhak, Lecture at Kalacakra Tantra, Switzerland, 1985.

8. Detlef Ingo Lauf, *Secret Doctrines of the Tibetan Book of the Dead*, Shambala, Boulder and London, 1977.

9. Lama Chime Rinpoche, 'The Three Kayas', *The Middle Way*, p. 113, vol. XLVII, no. 2, August 1972.

10. Dharmakaya: 'The universal principle of all consciousness, the totality of becoming and being is potentially contained – comparable to the infinity of space, which embraces all things and is the "conditio sine qua non" of all that exists'. Lama Govinda, *Foundations of Tibetan Mysticism*, Rider & Co., London.

11. Thinley Norbu, *The Magic Dance*.

12. Fremantle, verbal commentary on the Six Realms.

13. Lati Rinbochay, *Death, Intermediate State and Rebirth*, Rider and Company, London, 1977.

14. John Blofeld, *Mantras, Sacred Words of Power*, George Allen & Unwin Ltd, London, 1979.

15. Lawrence Blair, *Rhythms of Vision*, p. 130, Paladin (UK), 1976.
16. Eric Cheetham, Course on Sutra Teachings at the Buddhist Society Summer School, UK, 1984.

3 The Tibetan Medical Philosophy of Health

1. Dr Yeshi Donden and Lobsang Rapgay, 'An Introduction to Tibetan Medicine', *gSORIG* no. 1, 1980, Library of Tibetan Works & Archives, Dharamsala.
2. Dr Yeshi Donden and Gyatsho Tshering, 'What is Tibetan Medicine?', *An Introduction to Tibetan Medicine*, a Tibetan Review Publication, New Delhi, 1976.
3. T.J. Tsarong, *Fundamentals of Tibetan Medicine*, Tibetan Medical Centre, Dharamsala, 1981.
4. A further and deeper explanation of the nature of the Three Humours is given by Herbert V. Guenther in *The Life and Teaching of Naropa*, p. 170.
5. Theodore Burang, *Tibetan Art of Healing*, p. 25, Watkins, London, 1974.
6. Keith Dowman, *Sky Dancer*, Routledge & Kegan Paul, London, 1984, p. 246.
7. The ovum was not known in the past – this is a modern updating, Tibetan medicine being a continuously evolving process. The text of the bShad rgyud says 'menstrual blood' instead of ovum.
8. T.J. Tsarong, *Fundamentals of Tibetan Medicine*.
9. Dr Tenzin Choedhak, Lectures given in London at RIGPA in 1984.
10. Tenzin Gyatso, the Dalai Lama, *The Kalacakra Tantra*, p. 24, Wisdom Publications, London, 1982.
11. Lama Govinda, 'Conscious Expansion', *The Middle Way*, August 1971, pp. 79–80.
12. Elisabeth Finckh, 'The Theory and Practice of Tibetan Medicine', *Tibetan Review*, vol. 16, no. 4, New Delhi, April 1981.
13. Ven. Dr Trogawa Rinpoche, Lectures given in London at RIGPA in 1984.
14. Lecture given by Dr Lobsang Rapgay at the European School of Osteopathy, January 1985, and also p. XII of his book *Tibetan Therapeutic Massage*.

4 Disease

1. Ven. Dr Trogawa Rinpoche, Lectures given in London at RIGPA, 1984.
2. Ven. Dr Trogawa Rinpoche, Lectures given in London at RIGPA, 1984.
3. Ven. Rechung Rinpoche, *Tibetan Medicine*, Wellcome Institute of the History of Medicine, London, 1973.

4. Dr Tenzin Choedhak, Lectures given in London at RIGPA, 1984.
5. Terence Clifford, *Tibetan Buddhist Medicine and Psychiatry*, p. 98, The Aquarian Press, Wellingborough (UK), 1984.
6. Theodore Burang, *Tibetan Art of Healing*, p. 50.
7. Doctors Tenzin Choedhak and Trogawa Rinpoche, Notes taken at their lectures at RIGPA, London, 1984.
8. Terence Clifford, *Tibetan Buddhist Medicine and Psychiatry*, p. 94.
9. Terence Clifford, *Tibetan Buddhist Medicine and Psychiatry*, p. 94.
10. T.J. Tsarong, *Fundamentals of Tibetan Medicine*, Tibetan Medical Centre, Dharamsala, 1981.
11. 'The Arisal of Discussion', *gSORIG* No. 2, 1981, p. 36, Library of Tibetan Works & Archives, Dharamsala.
12. Doctors Tenzin Choedhak and Trogawa Rinpoche, Notes taken at their lectures at RIGPA, London, 1984.

5 Diagnosis

1. 'Ambrosia Heart Tantra', Chapter 4, p. 37, *The Root Tantra*, Library of Tibetan Works & Archives, Dharamsala, 1977.
2. Table from *Fundamentals of Tibetan Medicine*, Tibetan Medical Centre (now Institute), Dharamsala, 1981.
3. Dr Barry Clark, verbal comment.
4. Dr Lobsang Rapgay, see Appendix 1.
5. See Appendix 2.
6. Based on notes taken during lectures by Ven. Dr Trogawa Rinpoche in London, 1984.

6 Mind and Mental Disorders

1. Dr Lobsang Rapgay, *Mind and Mental Disorders in Tibetan Medicine*, p. 29 (published by the author).
2. Ven. Chögyam Trungpa Rinpoche, Introduction to *Glimpses of the Abhidharma*, p. 3, Prajna Press, Boulder, USA, 1978.
3. Terence Clifford, *Diamond Healing – The Buddhist Medicine and Medical Psychiatry of Tibet*, (University Microfilms International) Preface p. iii.
4. Dr Lobsang Rapgay, *Mind and Mental Disorders*, p. 40.
5. Terence Clifford, *Tibetan Buddhist Medicine and Psychiatry*, pp. 137–8.
6. Terence Clifford, *Tibetan Buddhist Medicine*, pp. 130–1.
7. Theodore Burang, *Tibetan Art of Healing*, p. 89.
8. Dr Lobsang Rapgay, *Mind and Mental Disorders*, p. 25.
9. Edward M. Podvoll, MD, *Protecting Recovery from Psychosis in Home Environments*, Maitri Psychological Services, Boulder, USA, 1984.

7 Ecology and Tibetan Medicine

1. Based on notes taken at Dr Tenzin Choedhak's lectures given in London, 1984.
2. John Davidson, MA, *Journal of Alternative Medicine*, February 1985, p. 7.
3. TMI (Tibetan Medical Institute) 'News-Letter', vol. 1, no. 2, December 1982.

8 Introduction to Treatment

1. Kesang Tenzin, 'Methods of Healing', in *An Introduction to Tibetan Medicine*, a Tibetan Review Publication, p. 68.
2. Dr Yeshi Donden, 'Methods of Treatment in Tibetan Medicine', *gSORIG* No. 1, Library of Tibetan Works & Archives, p. 9.

9 Behavioural Therapy

1. Rechung Rinpoche, *Tibetan Medicine*, Wellcome Institute for the History of Medicine, p. 59, also Berkeley, University of California 1973 and 1976.
2. Rechung Rinpoche, *Tibetan Medicine*, p. 216.
3. Leaflet on the Rinchen Tso-tru Dhashed (Moon Crystal Pill), TMI, Dharamsala.

10 Treatment

1. From course notes taken during Teachings given by Dr Yeshi Donden in London, 1978.
2. Thinley Norbu, *The Magic Dance*, p. 89.
3. *Fundamentals of Tibetan Medicine*, Tibetan Medical Centre, Dharamsala, 1981, p. 33.
4. Rechung Rinpoche, *Tibetan Medicine*, p. 64.
5. Kelsang Rapten, B.Sc. (Biochemistry), 'Tibetan Medicinal Plants and Their Relationship to Modern Chemical Activity' – tSorig No. 3, Library of Tibetan Works & Archives, p. 32.
6. 'The Ambrosia Heart Tantra', Library of Tibetan Works & Archives, 1977, pp. 18–22.
7. Now published as the *British Herbal Pharmacopoeia* by the British Herbal Medicine Association, London, 1971.

11 Introduction to Relating Tibetan and Western Holistic Medicine

1. Fritjof Capra, *The Turning Point*, Flamingo – Fontana Paperbacks, London, 1983, p. 21.

2. Fritjof Capra, *The Turning Point*, pp. 31–2.
3. Harold Saxton Burr, *Blueprint for Immortality*, Neville Spearman, London, 1972.
4. Jens Jerndal, 'The Field Resonance Approach in Medicine', *Expansion*, #2, 1983.
5. Rene Dubos, *The Mirage of Health*, George Allen & Unwin, London, 1960.
6. Fritjof Capra, *The Turning Point*.
7. Von Bertalanfy, L., *Problems of Life*, Harper, New York, 1960.
8. Jens Jerndal, p. 11.
9. Rein, Glen, 'Bioelectric Magnetism and Psychic Healing', *Light* 103(3), pp. 116–23, 1983.
10. McDonagh, J.E.R., FRCS, *The Universe through Medicine*, William Heinemann (Medical Books) Ltd, London, 1940.
11. Laurence, George, *Radiesthesia IV*, London, 1952.
12. Laborit, H. *Réaction Organique à l'Agression et Choc*, Masson et Cie, Editeurs, Paris, 1955.
13. Kaptchuk, Ted J. *Chinese Medicine – The Web that has no Weaver*, Rider, London, 1983, p. 14.

12 Western Herbal Medicine

1. Simon Mills, 'Herbal Medicine – the physiomedical perspective', *Journal of Alternative Medicine*, August 1983.
2. J.M. Thurston, 'Philosophy of Physiomedicalism', Indiana, J.M. Thurston, 1900.
3. Albert W. and L.R. Priest, *Herbal Medication*, L.N. Fowler & Co. Ltd, Romford (Essex), 1982.

13 Homoeopathy

1. Samuel Hahnemann, *Organon of the Rational Art of Healing*, 1st Edition, 1810, translated by C.E. Wheeler, Everyman's Library, p. 94.
2. Charles E. Wheeler, MD, BS, BSc. (London), *An Introduction to the Principles and Practices of Homoeopathy*, published by The British Homoeopathic Association, London, 1920, pp. 9–10.
3. W.E. Boyd, MA, MD, MBrit. IRE, 'Biochemical and Biological Evidence of the Activity of High Potencies', from *The British Homoeopathic Journal*, London, 1954, vol. xliv, no. 1, generally, but particularly pp. 7 and 42 (Microdoses).
4. Benoytosh Bhattacharya, *The Science of Tridosha*, Gotham Book Mart, New York, 1951.
5. Dr Barry Clark (Tibetan Medicine) (Dharamsala) – a verbal remark to the author.

14 Osteopathy I

1. Thomas G. Dummer and Andre Mahé, *Out on the Fringe*, Max Parrish, London, 1963, pp. 36–7.
2. T.G. Dummer, 'The Concept of Osteopathic Medicine', *St Bartholomew's Hospital Journal*, vol. LXX, no. 6, June 1975.
3. Denslow, J.S., 'An Analysis of the Variability of Spinal Reflex Threshold', *Journal of Neuro-Physiology*, 7:207/215, July 1944.
   Denslow, J.S. and Hassett, C.C., 'Central Excitatory State associated with Postural Abnormalities', *Journal of Neuro-Physiology*, S: 3293/402, Sept. 1942.
   Korr Irvin, 'The Physiological Basis of Osteopathic Medicine', The Post-Graduate Institute of Osteopathic Medicine and Surgery, New York.
   'Clinical Signifiance of the Facilitated State', American Academy of Applied Osteopathy Year Book, 1963. Selected Works.
   Korr, I., Denslow, J.S. 'Quantitative Studies of Chronic Facilitation in Human Motor Neurone Pools', *American Journal of Physiology*, 105: 229/238, Aug. 1947.
   Korr, I. 'The Neural Basis of the "Somatic-dysfunction"', *Journal of American Osteopathy*, Dec. 1947.
   Korr, I. 'The Emerging Concept of the "Somatic-dysfunction"', American Academy of Applied Osteopathy Year Book, 1963 (PO Box 1050, Carmel, California, USA).
4. Sutherland, W.G., 'Possibilities in Relation to the Basilar Articulations of the Cranial Bowl', 1929 in *Collected Writings of William Garner Sutherland, D.O., D.Sc. (Hon.)*, The Sutherland Cranial Teaching Foundation, USA, 1967.
5. Sutherland, W.G., 'Possibilities in Relation to the Basilar Articulations', p. 85.
6. Sutherland, W.G., 'Possibilities in Relation to the Basilar Articulations', p. 243.

15 Osteopathy II

1. Blavatsky, H.P., *The Secret Doctrine*, vol. 1, p. 2, Theosophical University Press, Pasadena, 1963.
2. Lauf, Detlef Ingo, *Secret Doctrines of the Tibetan Books of the Dead*, p. 89, Shambala, Boulder & London, 1977.
3. Capra, Fritjof, *The Turning Point*, pp. 26 8, 185–332, Flamingo – Fontana Paperbacks, London, 1982.
4. Guenther, H., *Life and Teachings of Naropa*, p. 165.
5. Sutherland, W.G., *Collected Writings*, p. 160.
6. Sutherland, W.G., *Collected Writings*, pp. 201, 243.
7. Sutherland, W.G., *Collected Writings*, p. 157.
8. An affectionate nickname for Dr A.T. Still, the founder of osteopathy.
9. Donden, Yeshi and Tshering, Gyatsho, 'What is Tibetan Medicine',

p. 7 of *An Introduction to Tibetan Medicine*, a Tibetan Review Publication, 1976.

10. Thinley Norbu, *The Magic Dance*, p. 89, Jewel Publishing House, New York, 1985.

17 Psychological Counselling with Buddha Dharma and Tibetan Medical Philosophy as a Basis

1. *Jataka Tales*, published by the Pali Text Society in 6 volumes, 1895–1907. Reprinted in 1981; bound in 3 volumes by Routledge & Kegan Paul, London.
2. John Walters, *Mind Unshaken*, p. 48, Rider & Co., London, 1961.
3. Keith Dowman, *The Sky Dancer – The Secret Life of the Lady Yeshe Tsogyal*, p. 147, Routledge & Kegan Paul, London, 1984.
4. Terry Clifford, *Diamond Healing – The Buddhist Medicine and Medical Psychiatry of Tibet*, p. 26, University Microfilms, USA, 1977.

19 Self-Help Through Tibetan Buddhist Philosophy and Medicine

1. Prof. Namkhai Norbu, *The Cycle of Day and Night*, p. 46, Zhang Zhung Editions, Oakland, California, 1984.
2. Dr Pema Dorjee, TMI News-Letter, June 1985, p. 3.
3. His Holiness Wangchuk Dorje, 'The Mahamudra Eliminating the Darkness of Ignorance', pp. 39–50.
4. Tarthang Tulku, 'Kum Nye Relaxation', Part 1, Preface, p. VIII.
5. Ven. Dr Trogawa Rinpoche, Notes of Teachings given at RIGPA, 1985.

Bibliography

Ayurvedic Medicine

Bhattacharya, Dr B., *The Science of Tridosha*, New York, Gotham Book Mart, 41 West 47th Street, New York 19, 1951.
Thakkur, Chandrashekhar G., *Introduction to Ayurveda* (Basic Indian Medicine), Bombay, Ancient Wisdom Publications, 1965.
Thakkur, Chandrashekhar G., *Ayurveda for You*, Bombay, Ancient Wisdom Publications, 1967.

Buddhism (Mahayana)

Suzuki, Daisetz Teitaro, *Outlines of Mahayana Buddhism*, New York, Schocken Books, 1963.

Buddhism (Theravadin)

Walters, John, *Mind Unshaken*, London, Rider & Company, 1961.

Buddhist Medicine

Birnbaum, Raoul, *The Healing Buddha*, London, Rider & Company, 1979.
Fromm, Erich and Suzuki, Daisetz T., *Zen Buddhism & Psychoanalysis*, London, Souvenir Press, 1974.
Norbu, Namkha'i, *On Birth and Life*, Naples, Shang Shung Edizioni, 1983.

Chinese Medicine

Kaptchuk, Ted J., *Chinese Medicine, The Web that has no Weaver*, London, Rider & Company, 1983.
Lavier, Jacques, *Les Bases Traditionelles de l'Acupuncture Chinoise*, Paris, Librairie Maloine S.A., 1964.
Veith, Ilza (translated by), *The Yellow Emperor's Classic of Internal Medicine*, London, University of California Press, 1966.

Herbal Medicine

Beach, W., MD, *The Reformed Practice of Medicine*, Birmingham (UK), 1859.

Cook, W.H., MD, *The Science and Practice of Medicine*, Cincinnati, 1897.

Lyle, T.J., 'Physio-Medical Therapeutics', *Materia Medica and Pharmacy*, Ohio, T.J. Lyle, 1897.

Mills, Simon, 'Herbal Medicine – the Physiomedical Perspective', *Journal of Alternative Medicine*, August 1983.

Priest, Albert W. and Lily, R., *Herbal Medication*, Romford, Essex, L.N. Fowler & Co. Ltd, 1982.

Thomson, Samuel, *New Guide to Health; or Botanic Family Physician*, Boston, 1835.

Thurston, J.M., *Philosophy of Physiomedicalism*, Indiana, J.M. Thurston, 1900.

Homoeopathy

Bhattacharya, Dr Benoytosh, *The Science of Tridosha*, New York, Gotham Book Mart, 41 West 47th Street, New York 19, 1951.

Boyd, W.E. MA, MD, MBrit. IRE, 'Biochemical and Biological Evidence of the Activity of High Potencies', *British Homoeopathic Journal*, vol. xliv, no. 1, 1954.

Hahnemann, Samuel, *The Organon of Rational Art of Healing*, London, Everyman's Library, 1810.

Mattei, Comte Cesar, *Vade Mecum de l'Electro-Homoeopathie*, Bologne, Imprimerie Maregiani, Rue Marsala, N4.

Vannier, Leon, Various Works on Homoeopathy, Paris, Gaston Doin et Cie.

Osteopathy

Burns, L., 'Pathogenesis of Visceral Disease following Vertebral Lesions', *Journal of the American Osteopathic Association*, Chicago, 1948, pp. 29–48.

Burns & Treat, 'Incidence of Certain Aetiologic Factors in Cardiac Disorders', *Journal of the American Osteopathic Association*, March 1953.

Cole, 'Somatico-Visceral Reflexes', *Journal of the American Osteopathic Association*, Feb. 1953 and *AAO Year Book 1954, Part 1*.

Coujard, Roger, *Régulation Neuro Végétative de la Croissance et de l'Equilibre Tissulaires*, Paris, Vigot Frères, 1957.

Decourt, Philippe, *Etudes et Documents* (Première Série), Editions Internationales Hesperis-Tangier – Les Phenomes de Reilly, 1951.

Denslow, J.S., 'An Analysis of the Variability of Spinal Reflex Threshold', *Journal of Neuro-Physiology*, 7: 207–15, July 1944.

Denslow, J.S. and Hassett, C.C., 'Central Excitatory State associated with

Postural Abnormalities', *Journal of Neuro-Physiology*, S: 393–402, Sept. 1942.

Dummer, T.G., 'The Concept of Osteopathic Medicine', *St Bartholomew's Hospital Journal*, vol. LXX, no. 6, June 1975.

Goldstein, M.J., Korr, I.M., 'Dermatonal Autonomic Activity in Relation to Segmental Motor Reflex Threshold', *Federal Proceedings*, 7: 67, 1948.

Korr, I.M., 'The Neural Basis of the Osteopathic Lesion', *Journal of American Osteopathy*, Dec. 1947.

Korr, I.M. 'Clinical Significance of the Facilitated State', *American Academy of Applied Osteopathy Year Book*, PO Box 1050, Carmel, California, USA, 1963.

Korr, I.M., 'The Emerging Concept of the Osteopathic Lesion', *American Academy of Applied Osteopathy Year Book*, PO Box 1050, Carmel, California, USA, 1963.

Korr, I.M., Denslow and Krems, 'Quantitative Studies of Chronic Facilitation in Human Motor Neurone Pools', *American Journal of Physiology*, 105: 229–38, Aug. 1947.

Krogman, 'The Scars of Human Evolution', *Scientific American*, 185: 54–7, Dec. 1951.

Laborit, H., *Réaction Organique à l'agression et Choc*, Paris, Masson et Cie, 1955.

Laborit, H., *Stress and Cellular Function*, Philadelphia, USA, J.B. Lippincott Co., 1959.

Lendrum, F.C., *The Pathological Physiology of the Upright Posture*, Studies of Medicine, Springfield, Ill., USA, Chap. 20, published by Charles C. Thomas, 1951.

Speransky, 'Experimental & Clinical Labor Pneumonia', *American Review of Soviet Medicine*, 2: 22–7, October 1944.

Frankstein, S.I., in *Science*, 106–242, Sept. 12, 1947.

Travell & Rinzler, *American Heart Journal*, 35: 248–51, March 1948.

Bigelow & Travell, *Psychosomatic Medicine*, 9: 353–63, Nov./Dec. 1947.

Lewis & Kellgren, *Clinical Science*, 4: 47–71, June 1939.

Head, Sir John, *Brain*, 16: 1–33, 1893. 17: 339–480, 1894.

McKenzie, *Symptoms & Their Interpretations*, Edition 2 (Paul B. Hoeber), NY, 1912, p. 204ff.

Sutherland, W.G., *Collected Writings of William Garner Sutherland, DO, DSc. (Hon.)*, The Sutherland Cranial Teaching Foundation, USA, 1967.

Tee, Dr D., Body Chemistry and Osteopathy, *Year Book of the Osteopathic Institute of Applied Technique*, Maidstone, Kent, 1960.

Verner, Weint and Watkins, J.R., G.W. and R.J., *Rational Bacteriology*, New York, H. Wolff, 1953.

Tibet

Gyatso, Tenzin, the 14th Dalai Lama, *Tibet, my Land and my People*, New York, Potala Corporation, 1977.

Harrer, Heinrich, *Seven Years in Tibet*, London, Pan Books, 1956.

Trungpa, Chögyam, *Born in Tibet*, New York, Penguin Books, 1971.

Tibetan Buddhism

Blofeld, John, *The Way of Power*, London, George Allen & Unwin Limited, 1970.

Blofeld, John, *Mantras, sacred words of power*, London, George Allen & Unwin Limited, 1977.

Csoma de Koros, Alexander, *A Grammar of the Tibetan Language*, Delhi, The Jayed Press, 1973.

Dowman, Keith (Translation and Commentary), *The Legend of the Great Stupa*, Emeryville, California, Dharma Publishing, 1973.

Dowman, Keith (Translation and Commentary), *The Aspiration of Kuntuzangpo*, Kathmandu, Diamond Sow Publications, 1981.

Dowman, Keith, *The Sky Dancer*, London, Routledge & Kegan Paul, 1984.

Fremantle, Francesca and Trungpa, Chogyam, *The Tibetan Book of the Dead*, Berkeley & London, Shambala Publications, Inc., 1975.

Govinda, Lama Anagarika, *Foundations of Tibetan Mysticism*, London, Rider & Company, 1960.

Govinda, Lama Anagarika, *The Psychological Attitude of Early Buddhist Philosophy*, London, Rider & Company, 1969.

Govinda, Lama Anagarika, *Psycho-cosmic Symbolism of the Buddhist Stupa*, Emeryville, California, Dharma Publishing, 1976.

Guenther, Herbert, *The Life and Teaching of Naropa*, London, Oxford, New York, Oxford University Press, 1963.

Guenther, Herbert, *The Tantric View of Life*, Berkeley, California, Shambala Publications Inc., 1972.

Gyatso, Tenzin, the 14th Dalai Lama, *Universal Responsibility and the Good Heart*, Dharamsala, Library of Tibetan Works & Archives, 1980.

Lati Rinpochay & Hopkins, Jeffrey, *Death, Intermediate State and Rebirth*, London, Rider & Company, 1979.

Lauf, Detlef Ingo, *Tibetan Sacred Art*, Berkeley & London, Shambala Publications Inc., 1976.

Lauf, Detlef Ingo, *Secret Doctrines of the Tibetan Books of the Dead*, Boulder & London, Shambala Publications Inc., 1977.

Ling-pa, Jigme (Translation and commentary by Ven. Tulku Thondup), *The Dzogchen Innermost Essence Preliminary Practice*, Long-chen Nying-thig Ngön-drö Dharamsala, Library of Tibetan Works & Archives, 1982.

Long-ch'en Rab-jam-pa, H.H. Dudjom Rinpoche and Beru Khyentze Rinpoche, *An Introduction to Dzog Ch'en – The Four-Themed Precious Garland*, Dharamsala, Library of Tibetan Works & Archives, 1979.

Norbu, Namkha'i, *The Cycle of Day and Night*, Zhang Zhung Edition, Oakland, California, 1984.

Norbu, Thinley, *Magic Dance*, New York, Jewel Publishing House, 1985.

Trungpa, Chögyam, *Meditation in Action*, London, Vincent Stuart and John M. Watkins Limited, 1969.

Trungpa, Chögyam, *The Myth of Freedom*, Boulder and London, Shambala Publications Inc., 1976.

Trungpa, Chögyam, *Glimpses of the Abidharma*, Boulder, Prajna Press, 1978.

Tucci, Guiseppe, *The Theory and Practice of the Mandala*, London, Rider & Company, 1961.

Wang-Ch'ug Dorje, the 9th Karmapa, *The Mahamudra*, Dharamsala, Library of Tibetan Works & Archives, 1978.

Wayman, Alex, *The Buddhist Tantras*, London, Routledge & Kegan Paul Limited, 1973.

Tibetan Medicine

Burang, Theodore, *Tibetan Art of Healing*, London, Robinson & Watkins Books Limited, 1974.

Clifford, Terry, *Tibetan Buddhist Medicine and Psychiatry – The Diamond Healing*, Wellingborough, The Aquarian Press, 1984.

Dash, Bhagwan, *Tibetan Medicine – Yoga Sataka*, Dharamsala (India), Library of Tibetan Works & Archives, 1976.

Dönden, Yeshi, *Health through Balance*, Ithaca, New York, Snow Lion Publications, 1986.

Dönden, Yeshi and Kelsang, Jhampa, *The Ambrosia Heart Tantra*, Volume 1, Dharamsala, Library of Tibetan Works & Archives, 1977.

Finckh, Elisabeth, *Foundations of Tibetan Medicine*, Volume 1, Bridge Street, Dulverton, Somerset, Robinson & Watkins Books Limited, 1978. Volume II, London, Robinson Books, 1985.

Dolma Khangkar, Ama Lobsang – Lady Doctor, lectures on Tibetan Medicine, Library of Tibetan Works & Archives, Dharamsala, 1986.

Massin, Christophe, *La Médecine Tibétaine*, Paris, Editions de la Maisnie, 1982.

Meyer, Fernand, *GSO-BA RIGPA. Le Système médical tibetain*, Paris, Editions du Centre National de Recherche Scientifique, 1983.

Norbu, Dawa (Edited by – a compendium), 'An Introduction to Tibetan Medicine', New Delhi, *Tibetan Review*, 1976.

Rapgay, Lobsang, *Tibetan Medicine – a holistic approach to better health*, Dharamsala (India), 1984.

Rapgay, Lobsang, *Tibetan Therapeutic Massage*, Dharamsala (India), 1985.

Rechung, Rinpoche, *Tibetan Medicine*, London, Wellcome Institute of the History of Medicine, 1973.

Rovere, Pierfrancesco, *Constituzioni e generalita nella tradizione medica tibetana*, Estratto da MINERVA MEDICA, vol. 77, no. 18, pp. 761–6, 28 April 1986.

Tarthang, Tulku, *Kum Nye Relaxation*, vols 1 & 2, Berkeley, California, USA, Dharma Publishing Co., 1978.

Tsarong, Jigme, Krakton, Jhampa Gyaltsen, Chompel, Lobsang, *Fundamentals of Tibetan Medicine*, Dharamsala (India), Tibetan Medical Centre, 1981.

Vitiello, Luigi, *Introduction to Tibetan Medicine*, Naples, Shang Shung Edition, 1983.

Various Authors (edited by), *Tibetan Medicine* (tSorig), Dharamsala, Library of Tibetan Works & Archives. Series: no. 1, 1980; no. 2, 1981; no. 3, 1981; no., 4, 1981; no. 5, 1982; no. 6, 1983; no. 7, 1983; no. 8, 1984; no. 9, 1985.

General

Broad, C.D., *Religion, Philosophy and Psychical Research*, London, Routledge & Kegan Paul, 1953.

Grant, Joan and Kelsey, Denys, *Many Lifetimes*, London, Gollancz, 1967.

Herrick, Judson C., *The Evolution of Human Nature*, Austin, University of Texas Press, 1956.

Jacquin, Noel, *The Theory of Metaphysical Influence: A Study of Human Attunements, Perception, Intelligence and Motivation*, London, Rockliff, 1958.

Glossary of Tibetan Words with their phonetic equivalents

Tibetan words which are already given in phonetical transcription are not listed here. Transliterated terms in Appendix 1 (G), which is for scholars, are also not included. The words are arranged in English alphabetical order, including Tibetan prefixes to ease the use of the glossary by the general reader for whom it is intended.

dbag–'dzin:	*dak-dzin*
bDud-rtsi'i sNying-po:	*Dutsi Nying-po*
bsam-bse'u:	*sam-say*
bshad rgyud:	*shey-gyu*
bsKa-ba:	*Ka-wa*
Byang-pa:	*Chong-pa*
'Byung-ba lnga:	*Jung-wa nga*
Chos-grags rGya-mtsho:	*Chur-drak Gyamtso*
dbu-ma:	*oo-ma*
'dod-chags:	*dur-chak*
dpyad:	*chay*
drag dpyad:	*drak-chay*
dug-bcom:	*duk-chom*
gSer-bzang Dri-med:	*Ser-zong Dree-may*
gSo-dpyad 'Bum-pa:	*So-chay Bum-pa:* ('*Bum*' to rhyme with 'wom' in 'Woman')
gti-mug:	*ti-muk*
'Jam dpyad:	*Jam-chay*
kha-ba:	*kha-wa*
khrag:	*trak*

khu-ba:	*khu-wa*
klu:	*loo*
lan/tshwa:	*len-tsa*
Legs-bshad Nor-bu:	*Lek-shey Norbu*
Man-ngag rgyud:	*men-ngak gyu* ('*ng*' sound as in 'singer')
mngar:	*ngar*
mNgon-mkhyen rGyal-po:	*Ngurn-khyen Gyel-po*
mTshan-legs Yongs-grags:	*Tsen-lek Young-drok*
Mya-ngan-med-mchog:	*Nya-ngen-may-chok*
nam-mkha':	*nam-kha*
Nyan-nyid rDo-rje:	*Nyen-nyee Dorjay*
Nyes-pa:	*nyay-pa*
Padma:	*Pema*
phyi-ma rgyu:	*chee-ma gyu*
rGyud bzhi:	*Gyu zhee*
Rig-pa'i Ye-shes:	*Rik-pay Yeshay*
rKang:	*kong*
rtsa rgyud:	*tsa gyu*
rtsub-dpyad:	*tsup-chay*
sDe-srid Sangs-rgyas rGya-mtsho:	*Day-see Song-gyey Gyamtso*
sGra-bdyang rGyal-po:	*Dra-yong Gyel-po*
Sha-kya Thub-pa:	*Shakya Thup-pa*
Shel gyi me-long:	*shel gyi may-long*
SKur:	*Kyur*
sMan-lha:	*Men-hla*
sna rdzong:	*na dzong*
srog-rlung:	*sok-lung*
tshwa-ba:	*tsa-wa*
Vaidurya sNgon-po:	*Vaidurya Ngurn-po*
Yan-lag brgyad-pa chen-po:	*Yen-lak gyey-pa chen-po*
Yid-las-skye:	*Yid-lay-kyey*
zhe-sdang:	*zhay-dong*
Zur mKhar-ba:	*Zur khar-wa*

Index